MENDING BROKEN SOLDIERS

MENDING BROKEN SOLDIERS

—

THE UNION AND CONFEDERATE PROGRAMS TO SUPPLY ARTIFICIAL LIMBS

—

GUY R. HASEGAWA

WITH A FOREWORD BY JAMES M. SCHMIDT

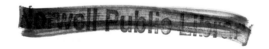
SOUTHERN ILLINOIS UNIVERSITY PRESS
CARBONDALE AND EDWARDSVILLE

15 14 13 12   4 3 2 1

Library of Congress Cataloging-in-Publication Data
Hasegawa, Guy R.
Mending broken soldiers : the Union and Confederate programs
to supply artificial limbs / Guy R. Hasegawa ; with a foreword by
James M. Schmidt.
     p. cm.
Includes bibliographical references and index.
ISBN 978-0-8093-3130-7 (cloth : alk. paper) — ISBN 0-8093-3130-6
(cloth : alk. paper) — ISBN 978-0-8093-3131-4 (ebook) — ISBN 0-8093-
3131-4 (ebook)
1. United States—History—Civil War, 1861–1865—Medical care.
2. United States—History—Civil War, 1861–1865—Technology.
3. Artificial limbs—United States—History—19th century. 4. Artificial limbs—Confederate States of America—History. 5. Amputees—Services for—United States—History—19th century. 6. Amputees—Services for—Confederate States of America—History.
7. Soldiers—Medical care—United States—History—19th century.
8. Soldiers—Medical care—Confederate States of America—History. I. Title.
E621.H33 2012
973.7'75—dc23   2012000923

Printed on recycled paper. ♲
The paper used in this publication meets the minimum requirements
of American National Standard for Information Sciences—Perma-
nence of Paper for Printed Library Materials, ANSI Z39.48-1992. ∞

To Betsy, David, and Stephen

CONTENTS

Gallery follows page 56

Visit http://www.siupress.com/product/Mending-Broken-Soldiers,5778.aspx for a list of Union soldiers and sailors supplied with artificial limbs by the U.S. government through mid-1866, and a list of Confederate soldiers for whom orders for artificial limbs were given through the Association for the Relief of Maimed Soldiers.

FOREWORD

———

T hough separated in their writing by almost 150 years, Oliver Goldsmith's "Deserted Village" (1770) and Katharine Tynan's "The Broken
Soldier" (1916) share important imagery. In his poem, Goldsmith writes
of "The broken soldier, kindly bid to stay . . . Shoulder'd his crutch and
show'd how fields were won." Tynan's, in title and verse, refers to "The
broken soldier . . . maimed and half-blind . . . One hand is but a stump and
his face a pitted mask." Note the word they use to describe the soldier:
not "crippled"; not "wounded" or "injured." *Broken.*

The choice is both poignant and fitting: wars do break things, especially
the men and women who fight them. From ancient times to the modern
day, humankind has devoted itself to perfecting the art and science of
destruction. At the same time, some people have devoted themselves to
"fixing" broken soldiers by crafting artificial legs, arms, eyes, and other
prosthetics. Pliny's *Natural History* recounts the exploits of Marcus Ser-
gius, a Roman general in the Second Punic War, who—having lost his
right hand in battle—"had a right hand made of iron for him" and returned to the battlefield. Medieval knights wore artificial limbs designed
by the blacksmiths who had built their armor. Modern war amputees
benefit from light composites and advanced electronics that make prosthetics ever more realistic and controllable.

At its heart, this book is about attempts to fix the "broken soldiers"
of the American Civil War. The unprecedented scale of that conflict—
in terms of armies raised, battles fought, technologies employed, and
soldiers wounded—resulted in no less than 60,000 amputations. Not
coincidentally, there was a large increase in inventive activity in prosthetics: patents for artificial limbs increased from less than thirty in the
previous decade to more than a hundred in the 1860s. "The havoc of war

has begotten a multitude of inventions to supply the place of amputated arms and legs," T. C. Theaker, the commissioner of patents, wrote in his annual report of 1865, adding a poignant note of a soldier who "sent a letter to the office written by an artificial arm and hand of his own invention."

The author—Guy R. Hasegawa—does a most admirable job in detailing the improvements in the mechanics, materials, and manufacture of prosthetics during the Civil War, from the simple (but still serviceable) peg leg to fully articulated artificial legs and arms with nearly natural motion and appearance. By the end of the war, Theaker could justly boast that "the United States are in advance of other countries at present in regard to this invention."

Still, the book is about much more than just the appendages themselves, and that is what makes it all the more original, interesting, and important. The author describes the political considerations of providing veterans with prosthetics at government expense; the continued professionalization of medicine as boards of experts examined and passed judgment on what limbs would be used and paid for; recriminations among inventors over patent infringement; the ethics of providing artificial limbs for prisoners of war; the lack of a native artificial limbs industry in the Confederacy—symptomatic of other industrial shortcomings—that handicapped its ability to provide for its own amputees; the inevitable encroachment of the "middle man"; and much more.

Allow me to say a word or two about the author: in regard to our shared interests in Civil War medicine and surgery, Guy Hasegawa has been a faithful correspondent and frequent collaborator, and my own research and writing have benefitted from his generosity and expertise. I'm honored that he asked me to write this foreword because he is also a dear friend. To any readers who might be inclined to discount what I say about him, I would ask that they take me all the more seriously *because* I know him; but read him for yourself: you will be treated to the results of thorough research backed by his expert knowledge of archival material, an entertaining narrative from his ever-able pen, and a refreshing economy of words owing to his eye as a professional editor.

In the end, it is not the empty sleeves of broken soldiers that define them, but—as Tynan wrote—"the soul they could not harm," which "goes singing like the lark."

James M. Schmidt

PREFACE

———

A mputation and the Civil War are immutably linked in the public imagination. The frequency of the operation, which occurred at least 60,000 times during the conflict, prompted citizens of the era to comment on how common it was to see young men returning home with an empty sleeve or empty pant leg. Today, a Civil War movie or reenactment seems incomplete if an amputee or amputation is not portrayed. Less generally recognized are the postwar programs that assisted military amputees by providing them with artificial limbs—this despite fine research on the topic by historians. Almost entirely absent, even among Civil War enthusiasts, is detailed knowledge of how amputees were helped *during* the war by the provision of artificial limbs. That story, told in this book, is one of dedicated individuals establishing programs from scratch—there were no templates for the wartime limbs programs—to furnish devices that they initially knew little about. The best of the limbs were marvels of craftsmanship and mechanical innovation and offered amputees the restoration of function and dignity.

My research for this book began with a volume titled *Record Book: Soldiers' Home Hospital and the Association for the Relief of Maimed Soldiers*, part of the War Department Collection of Confederate Records preserved by the National Archives and Records Administration (NARA) in Washington, D.C. Historians are blessed that masses of Confederate documents escaped destruction at the end of the Civil War and remain available for study. The survival of the records of the Association for the Relief of Maimed Soldiers (ARMS) is especially remarkable. ARMS, which supplied Confederate military amputees with artificial limbs during the war, was not a bona fide government organization, so its records would not ordinarily have been mingled with official documents. As luck would have it, the corresponding secretary for ARMS was Surgeon William A. Carrington, who was in charge of all army hospitals in Virginia. Carrington evidently directed his clerks to transcribe ARMS correspondence and reports on the empty pages of the official record book for Richmond's Soldiers Home Hospital. Furthermore, many ARMS-related documents not included in that ledger were also treated as official and reside elsewhere in NARA's collection.

It quickly became obvious that the ARMS story could be appreciated best only if accompanied by a parallel account of the Union program and with background information about artificial limbs themselves. The Union effort was administered by the surgeon general of the army, which suggested that its history could also be reconstructed from records at NARA. Indeed, the correspondence of the surgeon general was vital, but the army's and NARA's record-keeping practices resulted in relevant material being dispersed among various NARA record groups, including those of the Adjutant General's Office and U.S. Army Commands, and even to at least one other repository. I cannot claim to have examined all of the Union or Confederate documents pertinent to the topic, and there are gaps in the records I have recovered, yet what emerges is nonetheless a fascinating account.

As for the descriptions of the limbs and the companies making them, I relied heavily on pamphlets and other publications of the firms themselves. One maker in particular, Benjamin Franklin (B. Frank.) Palmer, was especially active in self-promotion and wrote often to the U.S. surgeon general, so if he seems to get more attention here than he deserves, it is because of the relative abundance of information about him. Many artificial-limb companies operated during the war, and to help readers keep track of them, brief descriptions of the firms that were important to this story are provided in appendix A.

The story of the limbs programs is intriguing in its own right and has much to offer readers with a general interest in the Civil War or the history of medicine. At another level, though, the account serves as a case study illustrating the vast differences between the Union and the Confederacy in industrial capacity and economic conditions. The aims of the programs were identical, and their administrators often arrived at similar means to meet their challenges, yet the particular difficulties faced by the Confederacy— the lack of a prewar Southern limbs industry and the Union naval blockade, for example—made for obstacles that could never be completely overcome.

The programs existed in the first place, of course, to assist military amputees, thousands of whom received artificial limbs. Lest readers lose sight of the individuals who sacrificed so much, Southern Illinois University

Press has posted lists of the soldiers and sailors who received a limb through the wartime U.S. program or who applied for a limb through the Confederate program. (Go to www.siupress.com for a link to the lists.)

Readers commonly wonder about the relevance of history to current events. In this instance, the connection is apparent. The conflicts in Afghanistan and Iraq are producing grim casualties among service members, many of whom can be assisted by artificial limbs. The commitment to provide this support to American military personnel started with the programs described in this book. One of today's major artificial-limb companies, in fact, was founded during the Civil War and furnished legs to Confederate amputees.

Thus, it is my hope that this book will tell a good story, provide insight into how the North and South differed in striving to attain the same goal, and prompt readers to reflect on the grievous wounds inflicted by war and how well-meaning people have tried to mitigate the resultant suffering.

Various individuals and organizations had a hand in making the publication of this book a reality. One of the project's earliest supporters was F. Terry Hambrecht, a long-time friend and expert in Civil War medicine, who provided information from his vast library and files as well as encouragement and advice. My good friend James M. Schmidt, who kindly contributed the foreword, is an accomplished Civil War researcher and historical author and helped me navigate my first solo venture into book publishing. Both Terry and Jim reviewed drafts of the book's chapters and provided valuable feedback. Sylvia Frank Rodrigue, acquisitions editor for Southern Illinois University Press, saw value in my book proposal and guided me through manuscript review, revision, and publication with patience and professionalism.

Michael Rhode of the National Museum of Health and Medicine in Washington, D.C., furnished historical photographs, and Alan Hawk of the same institution showed me artificial limbs in the museum's collection and provided photographs of them for study and inclusion in this book. Lori Eggleston and Terry Reimer of the National Museum of Civil War Medicine in Frederick, Maryland, supplied information from the museum's historical files and photographs of artifacts in its collection. Hanger Orthopedic Group in Austin, Texas, provided helpful material from company archives.

Finally, writing this book would not have been possible without the patience and encouragement of my wife, Betsy, and our sons, David and Stephen, who have been my faithful supporters since my first foray into Civil War research more than a dozen years ago.

MENDING BROKEN SOLDIERS

1

─────

MELANCHOLY HARVEST

It is not two years since the sight of a person who had lost one
of his lower limbs was an infrequent occurrence. Now, alas!
there are few of us who have not a cripple among our friends,
if not in our own families. A mechanical art which provided
for an occasional and exceptional want has become a great and
active branch of industry. War unmakes legs, and human skill
must supply their places as it best may.
        —Oliver Wendell Holmes, M.D., "The Human
                Wheel, Its Spokes and Felloes," 1863

On the evening of September 1, 1862, Major General Ambrose Powell
Hill sent his Confederate division forward to engage the enemy
at a position called Ox Hill, near Chantilly Plantation, Virginia. As Hill
described it, the battle commenced with "a heavy, blinding, rain-storm
directly in the faces of my men," and one of his brigades in particular,
that of Brigadier General Lawrence O'Bryan Branch, took heavy fire to
its front and flank. The casualties in Hill's division from that engagement
numbered 39 killed and 306 wounded. Among the latter was Captain
Walter W. Lenoir of the 37th North Carolina Infantry of Branch's Brigade.
"I was shot through the right leg about halfway between the knee and
ankle," Lenoir informed his mother, "the ball striking both bones and
breaking the leg. Just afterward a ball struck the same leg, taking off the
end of the toe and baring the shin bone between the other wound and
the knee." Lenoir's leg was amputated below the knee two days later.[1]

Rifle fire in another battle claimed a leg of Lieutenant William H. Baxter of the 113th Ohio Infantry. While advancing during the Battle of Ken-
nesaw Mountain on June 27, 1864, Baxter suddenly felt "a great shock like
the terrific jar of a peal of thunder close at hand. I took a step forward and
found my foot give way under me and I fell to the ground. At once I knew

I had been wounded. Immediately examining the wound, I found both bones of my leg smashed to pieces a few inches above the ankle." Baxter was taken to a field hospital, where his leg was amputated four inches below the knee, and then to a general hospital in Chattanooga. There, he "was awakened from a doze by a sound like water pattering upon the floor." It was blood from a fellow patient who had undergone a thigh amputation; the hemorrhage was stopped, but the man died soon afterward. On the stump of another amputee, "the flesh had drawn away, and shrunk back from the end of the bone, leaving it protruding quite a distance"; that man also died. "The sloughing away of the artery of an amputated leg" killed yet another patient, this one in the cot next to Baxter's.[2]

"The limbs of our friends and countrymen," observed physician Oliver Wendell Holmes, "are a part of the melancholy harvest which War is sweeping down with Dalhgren's mowing-machine and the patent reapers of Springfield and Hartford." That harvest included the appendages of some 60,000 soldiers, North and South—the actual number is unknown—who underwent amputation during the Civil War. Most had sustained one or more bullet wounds, typically from so-called minié balls fired from rifled muskets. These projectiles tended to shatter bone and damage the surrounding tissue considerably; surgeons were often left with no choice but to amputate.[3]

Wounds caused by artillery, although less common, also took their toll. The amputation purported to be the first of the Civil War, in fact, was performed after a six-pound solid shot struck the leg of a young Virginian named James Edward Hanger, who would soon come to play a major role in the Confederate artificial-limbs industry. Private Stephen D. Smith, part of the force assaulting the Confederate stronghold of Fort Wagner on Morris Island, South Carolina, was also felled by artillery. "I was hit," recalled Smith, a member of the 7th New Hampshire Infantry, "just as I was about to step down into the ditch in front of the fort. . . . I landed at the bottom of the ditch on my back, my left leg being under me and the left foot being up between my shoulders, the thigh being badly shattered by grape shot, and the wound was bleeding very fast." The quick-thinking Smith saved his own life by tying a makeshift tourniquet above the wound, and Confederate surgeons amputated at the thigh two days later.[4]

Smith, who was exchanged and survived the war, might have considered himself lucky. Union records show that the overall survival rate after amputation was about 75 percent but decreased the closer the operation was to the trunk. Soldiers having part of a foot removed, for example, had a 96 percent chance of survival, whereas only 17 percent of soldiers survived amputation at the hip joint. Statistically speaking, Smith's chance of surviving thigh amputation had been slightly lower than fifty–fifty.[5]

Amputation—usually performed while the patient was anesthetized with chloroform or ether—was the most common major surgical operation of the war. A skilled and experienced surgeon could perform the procedure in a few minutes. Speed was desirable, even when other patients were not awaiting surgery, because it helped minimize blood loss and the duration of anesthesia. Speed may also have contributed to the belief that callous army surgeons, eager to use the saw, resorted too often to amputation as the quick, convenient, and definitive treatment for a limb injury when they should instead have waited for the wound to heal itself or taken other more laborious steps to save the limb. Although some limbs were certainly amputated unnecessarily, some physicians of the time argued that more wounded soldiers would have survived had surgeons been quicker or more willing to remove mutilated limbs. The danger of not promptly removing a limb that had extensive bone or tissue damage was that an intractable infection would set in; if it did not spread and kill the patient, it could still cause chronic illness and incapacitation. How to prevent or treat infection—or that microbes were even involved—was not yet known. Infection was also practically inevitable after amputation but was usually of a severity more likely to allow recovery, and this knowledge led surgeons to consider amputation the lesser of two evils. To be sure, the complications of amputation could be fatal, as Lieutenant Baxter observed among the fellow amputees in his hospital ward.[6]

With some 45,000 survivors of amputation, the demand for artificial limbs was considerable, although not all the survivors were candidates. About 38 percent of Union amputation survivors, for example, had undergone removal of fingers or toes or part of a hand or foot, and in such instances, there might not be a particular desire or need for an artificial replacement if one could even be found. The absence of a stump—in cases of amputation at the shoulder or hip joint—made the fitting of a useful prosthesis difficult. Some amputations resulted in a stump without enough tissue covering the bone to allow the comfortable wearing of an artificial limb. Chronic infection of the limb might make the wearing of a prosthesis impossible or impractical. Finally, some soldiers simply preferred to go without.[7]

Most amputees would have agreed upon the attributes of the ideal artificial limb—ease and naturalness of motion, realistic appearance, durability, lightness, and affordability—regardless of why they wanted a prosthesis. A simple desire to ambulate without the inconvenience of crutches would seem reason enough, yet there often existed other underlying motives. Primary among them was a desire to return to a previous occupation or, if that was impossible, to at least earn a living. The majority of Civil War amputees, North and South, had been farmers, planters, or skilled laborers and needed adequate mobility to return to work. Professional men who had lost their dominant arm still needed the ability to write, which might be restored by the appropriate artificial arm and hand. Many recipients of artificial limbs, said one periodical, could "attend to business, and thus make their livelihood" but, if not for their prostheses, "would have been helpless cripples—a trouble to their friends, and a burden to themselves all their lives."[8]

Some veterans may have been proud to display their empty pant leg or empty sleeve as evidence of their patriotic sacrifice, a scenario romanticized by a Southern poet:

> I see the people in the street
> > Look at your sleeve with kindling eyes;
> And you know, Tom, there's naught so sweet
> > As homage shown in mute surmise.[9]

Other amputees found it important to disguise their disability as much as possible. "In higher social positions, and at an age when appearances are realities," noted Holmes, "it becomes important to provide the cripple with a limb which shall be presentable in polite society, where misfortunes of a certain obtrusiveness may be pitied, but are never tolerated under the chandeliers."[10]

Ten days after his amputation, Walter Lenoir wrote, "Dear mother I wish to say to you that I am entirely reconciled to bear my wounds and sufferings in the good cause of my country's independence and that viewed in that light I look upon them with entire content and cheerfulness." Lenoir had, perhaps, not yet realized the extent to which his loss would affect him. That awareness, thought diarist Mary Boykin Chesnut, had come to Confederate general John Bell Hood when she observed him seventeen months after his leg, injured at Chickamauga, was amputated. "Much he knows," wrote Chesnut, "of the tortures of that stalwart frame maimed and lamed." The amputee's tortures, according to a limb manufacturer, extended beyond "the mere privation of [the lost limb's] previous service. His affliction is to be estimated, morally, by his mortified and wounded sensibilities, and physically, by a long train of cruel sufferings." The physical problems included "disturbance of the balance between nutrition and assimilation, producing plethoric and apoplectic symptoms; the injurious effect of the use of crutches upon the circulation, the nervous system, the spine, the skeleton of the trunk, and the lungs."[11]

Wounded veterans did not necessarily care to share their ordeals with others or to be reminded of them. Because "mute surmise" was hardly the universal reaction to a missing arm or leg, amputees hoped that an artificial limb might help them avoid impertinent stares, comments, and questions. Even if public notice was not emotionally painful or embarrassing, it could nonetheless be a nuisance. The amputee, wrote a waggish veteran who had lost a leg, "is looked upon as public property, and is almost bored to death with questions, by the many curious strangers he meets." These might include queries such as "Did a cannon ball take it off?" and "Did you feel much pain?" "No one spares me," he complained, "except such as have been in the army themselves. Men, women, children, foreigners, fools and even negroes, subject me to this systematic torture."[12]

The ability to procure an artificial limb depended on one's location and means. At the outset of the war, limb manufacturers were numerous in the North, where they had been doing good business with victims of industrial, farming, and railroad accidents. Since there was no large-scale limb industry in the South, the Northern firms had counted Southern amputees among their customers. The commencement of the war dramatically curtailed trade between North and South, and Southern craftsmen began setting up shop to supply the customers that the battlefields were producing in ever-increasing numbers. The war began with Union and Confederate amputees being responsible for finding and paying for their own artificial limbs.

Some amputees turned to acquaintances or local craftsmen to make a crude "peg leg" because it was all they deemed necessary, could afford, or could obtain without inconvenient travel. Unless an amputee knew how to take the proper measurements, he had to incur travel and lodging expenses to visit a limb maker in person to have his stump examined and measured and then wait for the device to be custom-made. Walter Lenoir, now resigned from his North Carolina regiment, used a wooden leg fabricated by a brother until a more elegant one could be fashioned by a local carpenter named Montgomery, who had examined Northern-made specimens. Montgomery's device did not prove entirely satisfactory, although Lenoir supposed it was "as good as they make 'em,'" so he made another leg himself to wear around the farm, while saving "the Montgomery leg for riding and an occasional change." Lenoir and many novice limb makers seemed not to realize that good craftsmanship did not ensure that a prosthesis would be useful. The device also had to fit properly and be matched in design, function, weight, and other aspects with the particular needs and characteristics of the patient.[13]

Articulated (jointed) limbs from firms dedicated to their manufacture were widely available in the North—much less so in the South—but typically at great cost. A Palmer leg, probably the most celebrated model of the era, was usually sold for $150 in the North, a considerable sum for someone who had been receiving a private's pay of $13 a month. A Southerner, who might expect to pay $300 to $500 in inflated Confederate currency for a Confederate-made leg, was in even a worse predicament because soldiers' pay lagged so far behind the rate of inflation. One such soldier was Private Thomas Welch of the 9th Alabama Infantry, who underwent amputation after being shot in the knee at Chancellorsville. "I am in indigent circumstances," he stated, "and am unable to pay the price demanded for an artificial leg." Added to amputees' concerns was the fact that artificial limbs wore out and generally had to be replaced every several years.[14]

In some instances, an individual benefactor paid for an amputee's artificial limb. Orderly Sergeant John McKenzie of the 79th New York Infantry, shot twice in the leg at the first Battle of Bull Run, underwent amputation and "was furnished at the private expense of the Hon. Simon Cameron with an artificial limb." Other amputees were lucky enough to have friends and neighbors take up a collection to pay for a limb.[15]

Not only was Sergeant McKenzie saved the expense of a limb, he was also eligible for a government pension of $8 a month, to which congressional acts of July 22, 1861, and July 14, 1862, entitled him. The first act, which authorized the president to accept the services of up to 500,000 volunteers, provided volunteers who became disabled while serving the United States with the same benefits due to disabled members of the regular army; the provision was intended, in part, to encourage enlistments. The second act refined and clarified the first and set forth the particulars of the administration and payment of pensions. The acts, however, did not address the government provision of artificial limbs or provide enough compensation for individuals of lower military rank to afford them. Specific assistance for amputees first appeared in a congressional act of July 16, 1862, in which the modest amount of $15,000 was appropriated to purchase limbs for maimed soldiers and sailors. A robust program subsequently blossomed with the assistance of other appropriations and an abundance of manufacturers eager to get a piece of the government pie.[16]

Meanwhile, no analogous legislation occurred in the Confederate Congress, and Southern amputees were left to fend for themselves. Finally, in January 1864, a nongovernmental association, headquartered in Richmond, was established to procure and pay for artificial limbs for Confederate military amputees. This organization was probably the only Confederacy-wide relief society founded by civilians.[17]

The following chapters describe those wartime efforts to provide artificial limbs to men maimed in the service of their country. The Union program was marked by intense competition among numerous firms to become a government-approved supplier and the efforts of civilian and military physicians to select the most appropriate limbs from the many available. The Confederate program's administrators and manufacturers struggled to overcome the problems that vexed Southern industry in general: a shortage of established makers and a scarcity of money, skilled labor, and materials. Although the operations differed vastly in resources and organization, they shared the distinction of being run not by petty bureaucrats but by military surgeons of high standing who had amputees' interests at heart and wielded enough power and influence to move the programs along. The administrators of both programs devised remarkably similar methods to facilitate the provision of limbs and make manufacturers accountable for their quality. For all their pacific intent, the endeavors, especially in the South, came to involve a surprising array of military men best known for their battlefield exploits. Prominent politicians and other individuals of note also found themselves playing a role in the programs. As Dr. Holmes observed, the war's maimed were ubiquitous, and it was nearly impossible not to have an interest in them— personal, political, business, or otherwise.[18]

A proper understanding of the programs requires knowledge of the American limbs industry as it existed shortly before and during the war: who made the devices, how they were constructed, and the relationships among the various makers. This is an intriguing account in its own right—of mechanical ingenuity, bitter rivalry, and shrewd business positioning—and makes a fitting prelude to the story of the Civil War's artificial-limbs programs.

2

THE BEST SUBSTITUTES KNOWN TO ART

When surgery is a perfected science, and amputation—its op-
probrium—has ceased to be a common operation, these willow
and parchment counterfeits of good Christian legs will be of
less account; but till then there is no fear that *MESSRS. PALMER
& Co.*, will not be appreciated as benefactors by many unfortunate cripples and all their friends.

—*New York Times*, 1855

Out of ten men walking down the street, each wearing an artificial
leg, said the *American Medical Times* in 1862, "in nine we are more
liable to fix the disability upon the natural than the artificial limb." Testimonials of the era described limb recipients being able to walk, climb and
descend stairs, dance, or ride a horse with ease. "I suppose," wrote one customer to his limb maker, "you will scarcely credit when I tell you I skated
three hours last week—such, however, is the fact." A railroad conductor
reported that his artificial leg allowed him to perform activities such as
"jumping on and off at stations, passing quickly through the train from
one car to another, &c." A state-of-the-art artificial limb, when properly fit,
could indeed be a godsend to an amputee. Limb makers—engaged in an
innovative, growing, and exceedingly competitive business—created high
expectations and endeavored to supply devices that satisfied those hopes.[1]

The lineage of many artificial limbs of the Civil War can be traced to
the Battle of Waterloo in 1815, where an artillery projectile struck the leg
of British cavalry commander Henry William Paget, Lord Uxbridge, and
necessitated its amputation. Shortly thereafter, the nobleman, newly titled
the Marquis of Anglesey, asked one James Potts of London to supply an
artificial limb. Potts's design, said to be superior to others available at the
time, gave the Marquis great satisfaction and became known as the Anglesey leg. (Potts, who had lost one of his own legs, illustrated the oft-repeated

8

phenomenon of amputees manufacturing limbs.) Potts later took on an assistant named William Selpho, and the two worked together for eleven years. After Potts died, Selpho sailed to New York in 1839 to start his own business in "a country so rapidly advancing in the scale of nations." Selpho became a major manufacturer and remained so throughout the Civil War.[2]

One American user of the Anglesey leg was Benjamin Franklin Palmer—or B. Frank. Palmer, as he preferred to be called—whose leg was "ground off in a bark mill" when he was ten or eleven years old. Palmer, born in 1824, tried and was dissatisfied with "all the most approved artificial legs," including the Anglesey model—possibly made by Selpho—and resorted to fashioning his own out of a section of willow tree from his New Hampshire farm. In 1846, Palmer secured the first American patent for an artificial limb and began "venturing to expose [the invention] to the gaze of a scrutinizing public." Palmer's device first earned acclaim at the 1846 National Fair in Washington, D.C.[3]

In 1847, Palmer opened a manufactory at Meredith Bridge, New Hampshire. He later took on partners, moved the business to Springfield, Massachusetts, and established offices in Philadelphia and other cities; he even granted a manufacturing license to a firm in London, England. Among Palmer's employees and partners before the Civil War were men who later started their own companies and became business competitors. The excellence of Palmer's product and his company's position as an incubator of future rivals made him the central figure in the American artificial-limb industry during the mid-1800s. Contributing to his recognition were his ceaseless self-promotion and his equally persistent criticism of competitors, especially those who had once worked with or for him.[4]

Palmer's associates included Richard Clement, whom he met in 1846 and hired as one of his first workmen; by 1860, Clement had established his own company. Former Palmer workmen Benjamin W. Jewett and Darwin DeForrest Douglass each entered the field with his own limb manufactory. Erasmus Darwin Hudson, M.D., purchased an interest in Palmer's patents in the late 1840s, became a business partner, and directed Palmer's Springfield branch when Palmer left to run the Philadelphia office. In the early 1860s, Hudson started his own business furnishing "improved" versions of the Palmer limbs. Marvin Lincoln held an interest in Palmer's business in the late 1850s and was foreman in one of the branches before starting his own company, which specialized in artificial arms.[5]

The number of manufacturers emanating from just Palmer's shops reflected the overall expansion in the artificial-limbs industry—a phenomenon of the Northern states—in the years leading to and including the Civil War. Patents for prostheses also grew more numerous during the era. Palmer had the only two American patents for artificial limbs in the 1840s, and only six more were issued in 1850–54. The number grew to sixteen in 1855–59, thirty-nine in 1860–64, and sixty-two in 1865–69; no patents for these devices before or during the war were from states that became part of the Confederacy. Patent activity by itself, however, may underrepresent the era's inventiveness and enterprise, especially with regard to medical devices, since various factors, such as altruism, may have discouraged some inventors from patenting their designs.[6]

One probable influence on patent activity was the set of beliefs expressed in the code of ethics of the American Medical Association, which stated that it was "derogatory to the dignity of the [medical] profession to resort to public advertisements . . . to boast of cures and remedies, to adduce certificates of skill and success, or to perform any other similar acts." Such were the acts of practitioners considered quacks by mainstream physicians, acts that were regarded as "highly reprehensible in a regular physician." It was also, said the code, "derogatory to professional character . . . for a physician to hold a patent for any surgical instrument or medicine." A common sentiment of the time was that a physician should not "monopolize or conceal the results of his observation, knowledge, or skill." One professor of surgery even equated the patenting of medical inventions with charlatanism, whether the inventor was a physician or not. Of the major limb manufacturers of the time, only two—Douglas Bly and the aforementioned E. D. Hudson—were physicians. Bly patented his limb designs whereas Hudson did not. Hudson "endeavored to combine all that is truly desirable and useful in limbs . . . without applying for patents or seeking the monopoly of any excellence," although he did purchase an interest in Palmer's patents. Those manufacturers who did have patents devoted considerable attention to publicizing and protecting them.[7]

The growing need for limbs, said one manufacturer, arose from "the rapid expansion of railroad systems . . . the increase of manufactories that employed ponderous and dangerous machinery; the invention and introduction of agricultural implements, such as mowing machines, reapers, threshing machines; the opening of mines, and the conversion of great forests into timber." Such activities, he continued, "had their distressing effect in dismembering the human body." In 1860, *Scientific American* told its readers that "the number of persons in the community who have lost a limb would surprise any one not familiar with the statistics" and that "the aggregate amount of almost any article in use in a great nation is immensely larger than would be anticipated." The Civil War, of course, created large numbers of new customers and a business climate ripe for enterprising limb makers. As one periodical said in 1863 of a supplier, "In these days of demand for Artificial Legs, if Mr. [Charles] Stafford [producing a leg patented by O. D. Wilcox] does not amass a fortune, it will not be because he does not sell a good artificial limb." Adding to the lucrativeness of the business was the likelihood that some customers, dissatisfied with their current prosthesis, would be seeking another and the fact that artificial limbs wore out and had to be replaced from time to time.[8]

Contemporary with the growth in the artificial-limb industry was the rise of a specialty called mechanical surgery, which encompassed "the treatment with apparatus of mutilations and deformities" and included the design and fitting of devices such as trusses and artificial limbs. The *American Medical Times* opined that "the Mechanical Surgeon, or the 'Surgeon Artist,' to use an elegant phrase, must be a thoroughly educated physician as well as an inventive genius"; being an amputee—a condition common to so many makers—was not enough of a qualification. Instead, the specialty required "accurate knowledge of anatomy, of physiology, and of surgery." The periodical continued by condemning "on all occasions, and under all circumstances, the uneducated pretenders in this department of surgery, who throng our cities, and trumpet their wares in every market." The physician limb-manufacturers Hudson and Bly embraced these points in their promotional efforts, with Hudson proclaiming his extensive experience in the field and Bly billing himself as "anatomist and surgeon." Bly stated that limbs that preceded his own had been made entirely by "common mechanics and *those who have undergone amputation*, but who have little or no knowledge of anatomy"[9]

Nonphysician limb makers countered by touting their own suitability to produce prostheses. Palmer, in particular, believed himself at least as qualified in mechanical surgery as a physician, or tried to give the impression that he was. He called himself a "surgeon artist"—the "elegant phrase" mentioned by the *American Medical Times*—cited his long experience, second only to Selpho's in the United States, and published advice about the amputation sites along a limb that were most likely to result in a stump well suited for a prosthesis. After he received the honorary degree of doctor of laws, he started inserting "Dr." in front of his name in advertisements, often without indicating the basis for that title. James A. Foster, who started a limb company in 1864, dismissed the devices made by "doctors, lawyers [a probable reference to Palmer] and common mechanics" and claimed that his own qualifications—true expertise as a mechanic, a stint working for an established maker, and being an amputee—were ample. However strongly some physicians may have resented them, limb makers who were not medically trained seemed to have little difficulty getting prominent medical men to endorse their products.[10]

The typical articulated artificial limb of the time was constructed of willow wood hand-shaped to the contours of the human extremity and hollowed to lighten the device, receive the stump, and enclose the internal mechanism. Willow was not only light, strong, resistant to warping, and unlikely to irritate the stump, it also "approaches in longitudinal resiliency as near as may be to bone, and produces less jar than more solid material." Palmer reported seasoning his lumber for three years, much as was done for wood used in the manufacture of pianos. "The hollowing-out of the interior," reported one factory observer, "is done by wicked-looking blades and scoops at the end of long stems." For amputations below or at the knee, the artificial limb was usually hinged to an upper section, often made of leather, that laced around the thigh and prevented the device from slipping off the stump. Devices for above-knee amputations were often held in place by straps that looped over the shoulders or attached to a waist belt.[11]

Most models required individual fitting, although some designs were adjustable to fit patients and stumps of various sizes. It was generally thought best that the socket that received the stump "should be made of solid material, susceptible of a high degree of polish, and admitting of being accurately carved to fit the inequalities of the stump." This fit was accomplished after careful measurement of the stump and sometimes required the making of a cast. "No matter what may be the excellence of a leg in other respects," said one manufacturer, "*if the socket does not fit the stump,* the leg is worthless. It is *worse* than worthless. It becomes an instrument of *torture,* causing irritation, soreness, swelling and extreme suffering." A new stump shrank in the weeks after amputation, and ensuring a good fit depended in part on waiting for the stump's dimensions to stabilize.[12]

Manufacturer Amasa Abraham Marks experimented with a flexible leather socket that could be tightened or loosened to accommodate a stump that had changed in size, but he found that the material "did not possess the necessary rigidity to permanently oppose the weight of the wearer." Furthermore, "the leather or its lining would absorb the perspiration and become offensive, and worse still, by reducing the socket, the joints would be thrown out of line." Marks found that rawhide proved no better, and he abandoned the flexible socket before the war. The Wilcox leg used a "sack . . . made of any suitable material" as a socket; this design would seem to have presented many of the problems mentioned by Marks. Methods of providing air flow for the socket included drilling ventilation holes in the wooden leg piece and forming the socket of wire gauze. Odor could be a problem with wooden limbs. According to Hiram A. Kimball and Andrew J. Lawrence, who made their limbs of vulcanized rubber, "a wooden leg worn half a dozen summers with feverish perspiration soaked into the pores of soft porous wood there souring and drying makes it almost *insufferable* to repair, worse as a *companion*."[13]

The exterior of a carved wooden limb was typically enveloped with calfskin—possibly prepared as parchment—or similar material; one manufacturer said that the limb's form was "covered with a green calfskin dried and contracted on." According to a panel of surgeons, "no limb ought to be accepted, as reliable, which has sheep skin substituted for the raw calf, as a covering to the wood. . . . sheep skin soon rots, cracks, and peels off, thereby rendering the limb comparatively worthless." The covering used by Palmer—he reported using "delicate fawn skin" on his artificial arm—was attached with a waterproof cement. Bly described his limbs as being "enameled with the most delicate tinted flesh-colored enamel, shaded to suit each particular case."[14]

Cork, which was much too fragile to be employed in major structural components, was occasionally used as a covering or lining, which might account for artificial legs commonly being called "cork legs." Some makers fashioned the primary portions of their limbs out of materials other than wood, including steel, corrugated brass, vulcanized rubber, and "imperishable raw hide." An early design of John S. Drake employed a framework constructed partially of whalebone. Some makers—Dieterick W. Kolbe and William Selpho, for example—constructed arms out of leather. Edward Cotty made his artificial hand of German silver, an alloy of copper, nickel, and zinc.[15]

One of the more unusual designs—patented by George W. Yerger and often called the Ord leg because of Yerger's business partnership with John F. Ord—was a "skeleton" constructed of thin metallic ribs and hoops. Another novel limb was designed by amputee George B. Jewett of Salem, Massachusetts, and called the Salem leg to avoid confusion with the design of the evidently unrelated Benjamin W. Jewett. The Salem leg's major support was a central length of wood constituting an artificial tibia; this contrasted with most other legs, whose main support was a circumference of hollowed wood. The Salem mechanism was enclosed by a leather cover, which was laced in the back and stuffed with hair to give the limb a contour more or less like that of a natural leg.[16]

Joints were of various designs—ball and socket, hinge, and mortise and tenon, for example—and bolts at the knee and ankle joints could be made of iron, steel, brass, or vulcanized India rubber operating in bearings of similar material or in wood. The interior mechanisms governing the movement of the joints—such as making the heel go up and down in response to the bending or straightening of the knee—included cords of catgut or linen thread and springs of India rubber, steel, or brass. An artificial leg, said one physician, received its motive power "from the stump, and transmits it to the cords and springs, the latter probably contributing a very little through their elasticity." Pads between opposing surfaces helped prevent noise and often consisted of leather, buckskin, felt, or caoutchouc (rubber). Joints loosened by use could sometimes be tightened by wearer-accessible screws.[17]

One of the more contentious issues among designers was whether the ankle joint should have side-to-side motion. Such motion, absent in most artificial legs, was allowed to some extent by the play in Selpho's ankle joint and was a distinctive feature of the limb manufactured by Bly, who constructed his ankle as a "ball of polished ivory, plying in a socket of vulcanized rubber." Bly claimed that lateral ankle motion allowed the wearer to walk more easily along the side of a hill or inclined plane and to negotiate irregularities, such as small stones, in his or her path. Furthermore, contended Bly, his ankle joint required "no oil, a fact of no little importance, as those will testify who have worn legs with metallic joints, and been obliged to carry pocket oil cans." Among manufacturers who scorned Bly's design was Benjamin W. Jewett, who dismissed lateral ankle movement as "very pretty in theory" but "humbug" and "worse than useless in practice." He argued that side motion of the ankle was "under control of the will" in a natural limb but not in an artificial limb. Thus, the user of a device with lateral ankle motion would have his foot "turn in or turn out without his knowledge, and every step he takes is liable to throw him from his center of gravity." The desirability of lateral ankle motion remained unsettled among physicians who studied the question. Another notable departure in design was introduced in midwar by A. A. Marks, who sold an artificial leg with a solid rubber foot. The rubber's pliability, he maintained, allowed for elimination of the ankle and toe joints altogether.[18]

Although even a simple peg could restore some mobility to a patient who had lost a leg, designing a functional and esthetically acceptable arm and hand proved more challenging. An artificial arm ending in a hook might be somewhat useful but was inelegant and likely to draw unwanted attention. Among the designs with natural looking hands were those that featured movable fingers capable of grasping objects such as pens, forks, or reins and had ingenious and complex mechanisms operating their actions. One inventor explained how the movements were controlled: "Artificial arms as now used are operated by artificial tendons, ligaments, muscles, or straps, and the movements of the fingers are produced by movements of the arm, or upon straps passing around different parts of the body, or upon straps extending from the arm and operated by the other or natural hand." Thus, it was common for an artificial arm to be held on the stump by a strap that wound around the base of the opposite arm at the shoulder. Movement of that shoulder would change the tension on the strap, which was connected to a mechanism of cords, springs, levers, and pulleys that would flex or extend the fingers in unison. Palmer's elaborate design included fully articulated digits and a mechanism that could easily lock the hand closed or relax its grip. Other prominent makers of arms with movable fingers included Selpho, Kolbe, and Henry A. Gildea. Kolbe's limb and others could be fit with a hook or "tools of any suitable character" in place of the hand.[19]

The complex mechanisms of movable fingers were likely to get out of order, so some manufacturers advocated simpler, cheaper designs. Marvin Lincoln, the former Palmer associate, designed a hand that could hold an object placed between its immovable fingers and spring-loaded thumb. Lincoln's arm for above-elbow amputations could hang free or be locked with the elbow flexed to about a right angle, in which posture the user could, for example, clasp a bundle against his body. The natural hand was needed to operate a button to unlock the elbow. The hand on this model, too, could be replaced by a hook or other implement. In describing the sturdiness of his design, Lincoln reported that "it has been used to knock down men and horses, *though it is not recommended for such purposes.*" A. A. Marks produced a solid rubber hand pliable enough to hold a pen or other object placed in it. "It is as useful as any hand invented," said Marks, "which is not probably saying much in its favor, as no art yet shown, if it ever will, can compare with 'nature's handiwork.'"[20]

Patients who had suffered an injury to a limb bone without amputation did not need an artificial limb but might qualify for another type of device. In certain situations, surgeons elected not to amputate but to remove (excise or resect) the damaged section of bone instead and "spare the limb." Without the contiguous bone, though, the limb lost much of its strength, mobility, and function. E. D. Hudson was a pioneer in the design of an "apparatus for resection." As he described it, "To supply lost leverage, to give rigidity to the muscles, to restore the functions of flexion, extension, pronation and supination—impaired by wounds of the muscles or motor nerves—and leave the arm in a condition favorable to the reproduction of bone, and possible reunion, are the objects sought and obtained by this apparatus." For one patient who had undergone resection of the elbow, and in whom "three inches of the arm [was] composed exclusively of soft tissues," the apparatus consisted of "an enveloping aponeurosis [fibrous membrane] for the arm and forearm, to prevent the displacement of muscles, extending from the shoulder to the elbow, and thence to the wrist, united longitudinally by clasps, and supplied with [an] . . . articulation at the elbow." Flexion, extension, and rotation were assisted by "elastic rubber bands, attached to the apparatus by cords, and passing over . . . pulleys." Without the apparatus, the patient could do nothing with his arm, his forearm being "pendant and entirely invalidated [*sic*]," but seventy days after receiving the device, he could lift "a dumb-bell and a bucket of water to his head." Hudson speculated that "with [the apparatus's] introduction, the only objection to resection—uselessness of the mutilated arm—is obviated, and this operation will be extensively substituted for amputation."[21]

Limb makers displayed their wares at exhibitions and fairs in hopes that favorable showings—the entries were judged by panels of experts—would help separate them from their competitors. Thus, after his initial success at the National Fair in Washington, D.C., in 1846, Palmer moved on to successful exhibitions at the American Institute (New York), Massachusetts Charitable Mechanic Association, Connecticut Medical Society, New York Agricultural Society, Salem (Massachusetts) Charitable Mechanics' Association, Middlesex (Massachusetts) Mechanic Association, Franklin Institute (Philadelphia), Metropolitan Mechanics' Institute (Washington, D.C.), and Maryland Institute. Palmer also won the prize medal at the 1851 Great Exhibition in London. Other manufacturers at U.S. exhibitions included Selpho, James W. Weston, Bly, Lincoln, Yerger and Ord, Benjamin W. Jewett, and Marks. Although panels may have had some basis for comparing limbs for cleverness of design or elegance of finish, it is unclear how they were able to judge their durability, comfort, and naturalness of motion.[22]

Advertisements for limbs appeared in newspapers, popular periodicals, and medical journals. Many manufacturers also distributed pamphlets that described their products and services, listed the prizes garnered at exhibitions, and provided endorsements from physicians and testimonials from patients. According to an expert on Philadelphia manufacturers, Palmer was "so enterprising in making his inventions and facilities known" that saying more about him was unnecessary. "We can therefore proceed," he continued, "to notice some of the excellent manufacturers whose modesty is their chief fault." Those makers included Mason W. Matlack (yet another amputee), who succeeded Yerger and Ord in making their steel-skeleton limb, and the aforementioned Clement, Gildea, and Kolbe. Modest as these individuals may have been in comparison with Palmer, they were hardly reluctant to advertise.[23]

Many of the promotional themes were influenced by the relationships between Palmer and his former employees and partners. Manufacturers who had been associated with Palmer used his considerable prestige to enhance their own standing. Richard Clement referred to his long experience as foreman of "the largest [artificial limb] establishment of its kind," without mentioning Palmer as the company's head, and took credit for making the limbs acclaimed at London's Great Exhibition, again without mentioning that the devices were of Palmer's design. D. DeForrest Douglass claimed to have been "for several years the best workman of Palmer & Co." E. D. Hudson cited not only his years with Palmer but also the accolades accorded Palmer-model limbs as if he deserved the credit.[24]

Palmer grew increasingly indignant at the boldness of his former associates. Shortly before the war, he declared that, with one exception, infringements on his patents had been insignificant. The single important violator, he said, and one he tried to prosecute "for his piracy" was former workman Benjamin W. Jewett, "who fled from place to place at Mr. Palmer's approach, thus manifesting a consciousness of the dishonesty of his use of the invention." This "second-rate workman," said Palmer of Jewett, "never could gain my confidence or that of my first assistant, as he never produced a creditable limb." Palmer was still pursuing Jewett in 1862, by which time patent violations were, at least in Palmer's view, more problematic and merited disclosure in his literature; in one pamphlet, Palmer reported that Jewett had been arrested for patent violation and was "under heavy bonds." Former partner Hudson "cut from us both," said Palmer in 1862 in reference to himself and his remaining "honorable" partner, "and is now piratically trespassing upon my rights." Palmer commenced a suit against Hudson in 1861 but declined to proceed upon learning that Hudson was dangerously ill. Hudson countered by asserting in his pamphlets that he still rightfully possessed the interest he had purchased in Palmer's invention and had devoted his efforts while working with Palmer entirely to the good will of the company. Palmer's scorn for D. DeForrest Douglass peppered a published exchange that started with a claim that Douglass's limb was superior to Palmer's. Palmer responded that Douglass had been a mediocre workman at best—hardly "the best," as Douglass had claimed—and that his product was "almost an *exact copy* of the Palmer leg" in outward appearance and its only merit was taken from Palmer's design.[25]

The intense competition among manufacturers led them to insert into their promotional literature warnings to beware of imitators. Selpho cautioned readers as early as 1842 against makers pretending to produce the Anglesey leg. "Mr. S. introduced the article into this country," one of his advertisements stated, "and the mechanical principle upon which the peculiarity of the Leg depends, is known only in the United States to himself." Palmer alerted customers to manufacturers who were violating his patents and even threatened patients who used unauthorized copies. "A patentee has the same legal right to proceed against the user as against the vender of a patented article," said Palmer. "Most deeply should we regret," he continued, "to subject any person to any trouble or expense who had thus unknowingly purchased a limb which he had no legal right to use, and for this reason we feel it obligatory on us to caution the public against the imposition of infringers." Bly was more blunt in his literature: "Let it be remembered that each and every device herein described, is patented to me in the United States, England and France; and that whoever manufactures one of them within these countries, does it at his peril; also, that whoever uses one, incurs the same risk, unless he purchases it of me."[26]

Endorsements from prominent physicians added credibility and respectability to manufacturers' literature. Bly cautioned customers in 1861 to examine these statements closely: "Many surgeons who now recommend this [Bly's] leg, formerly recommended the Palmer Leg or others, which are out of date since this invention, but the makers still publish the old certificates, and very cunningly leave off the dates. No comment is necessary." As if to prove that imitators were rampant, D. DeForrest Douglass duplicated Bly's warning almost verbatim in 1865: "Surgeons who have formerly recommended other Legs are now recommending my invention. . . . But the manufacturers still continue to publish the old testimonials, given *before* my limb was introduced to the Profession, leaving off the date. Comment is unnecessary." Bly, at least, was correct, as illustrated by endorsements by eminent surgeon Valentine Mott. An 1851 endorsement by Mott appeared regularly, usually undated, in Palmer's promotional material. Selpho also featured an undated endorsement by Mott: "Best of all is the proof of those who wear them [Selpho's legs]. . . . Some of my friends, whom I have mutilated, inform me that they are superior to all others." Bly published a dated statement from Mott attesting to the superiority of Bly's leg over Palmer's. Dated statements from Mott approved Hudson's involvement in mechanical surgery and praised George B. Jewett's Salem leg.[27]

During the war, manufacturers were quick to identify the prominent military men among their customers. Palmer, for example, described his supplying Union general Oliver O. Howard with an arm and published a testimonial from General Daniel E. Sickles, who purchased a Palmer prosthesis after he lost a leg at Gettysburg. Testimonials from common soldiers also appeared, such as one given to A. A. Marks by William Deitz, formerly of the 29th New York Volunteers. Deitz had a rubber Marks foot installed on his artificial leg and "was very much pleased with the change" and wanted "no more to do with any of the confounded complicated and clattering wooden feet with their usual fixings." George W. Roberts of the Veteran Reserve Corps wrote to Richard Clement of his delight with his new leg and reported "dancing around on my pins as brisk as ever."[28]

The majority of published testimonials appeared as letters from civilian men and women who described how well they were getting along. Some reported casting aside the limb of a competitor—often Palmer, if one was named—and finding the advertiser's device much more satisfactory. Some of Selpho's promotional literature contained reproductions of handwritten letters submitted by customers wearing his artificial arm and hand. As to the value of such statements, a committee of surgeons that met shortly after war concluded that "no reliance was to be placed upon the value of published testimonials. . . . we feel constrained to caution the public against being influenced by such documents, and to enter our protest against the freedom with which such testimonials are usually given. . . . the testimony . . . was as strong in favor of the worst as the best, each being convinced of the superior merit of the patent which he wore." Testimonials nevertheless constituted a major component of promotional material and—because they appeared to be spontaneously offered by regular people—lent credence to manufacturers' claims of superiority.[29]

Amputees had ample reason to think that the available artificial limbs would serve them well, but lest their hopes grow too lofty, one surgeon cautioned that even the best device was "but a poor substitute for the natural member." An artificial leg, he continued, was "dependent on its gravity, the pressure of the body above, the action of the stump, the elasticity of the springs, the tention [sic] of cords or tendons, and the formation of its joints, for action more or less resembling those of the natural organ." This circumspect view went on: "It will wear out, and become deranged in its mechanism by violent or improper use. Care and patience is required in learning its action, and in accustoming the stump to weight and pressure." Nevertheless, the physician concluded, "from the start it will have the appearance of the natural leg, be a support to the body in standing, [and] assist in walking." And whatever the limitations of an artificial leg, declared another physician, "it is a vast improvement upon canes, crutches, and 'peg legs.'"[30]

Clearly, amputees could not expect perfection, but they could reasonably hope for a prosthesis that would allow them to ambulate, return to work, and avoid impertinent stares. It was with such goals that Union and Confederate organizations strove to supply war amputees with artificial limbs.

3

―――

NOBLE CHARITY

The Government, saved by the gallant United States troops . . . ,
should consider it a small part of its great duty to its mutilated
defenders, to restore, to the utmost extent possible, their comfort and usefulness, by supplying the *best artificial limbs.*
—B. Frank. Palmer, *Report of the Great
National Benefaction,* 1868

The group of physicians invited to gather in New York City on August 20, 1862, was a particularly distinguished one: career military
men such as surgeons Richard Sherwood Satterlee (U.S. Army medical
purveyor for New York) and Benjamin Franklin Bache (director of the
Naval Laboratory in Brooklyn and great grandson of Benjamin Franklin); and renowned civilian surgeons Valentine Mott and William Holme
Van Buren (Mott's son-in-law) of New York, Samuel D. Gross and Joseph
Pancoast of Philadelphia, and J. Mason Warren of Boston. Army Surgeon
General William A. Hammond had asked these men "to determine what
kind of Artificial Limbs should be adopted for the use of mutilated soldiers," and now most of them were assembled in Satterlee's office at the
corner of Greene and Broome Streets to begin the task.[1]

Five weeks earlier, on July 16, the U.S. Congress had appropriated
$15,000 for the purchase of artificial limbs for military amputees and
charged Hammond with administering the funds. It is unclear exactly
when the idea of furnishing limbs at government expense arose. Limb
manufacturer B. Frank. Palmer said that his knowledge of the country's
indebtedness to its wounded defenders prompted him in 1861 to recommend the measure to the Reverend Henry Whitney Bellows, president of
the U.S. Sanitary Commission, and to the surgeon general. They approved
of the suggestion but saw no way to implement it, so Palmer "called the attention of influential members of congress to the subject." The *American*

Medical Times suggested the furnishing of limbs as early as December 1861 as a way to reduce pension payments. Limbs, said the periodical, could make "many an idle pensioner capable of self-support" and "would be an economy in Government" while giving "to society many an active and useful member who would be otherwise a burden upon the public." Congress may have been spurred not only by economic and humanitarian concerns but also by the belief that the appropriation might make enlisting in the army more palatable; such was one of the motives behind pension legislation enacted about a year earlier.[2]

Also unclear is how Hammond, who had been surgeon general only since April 1862, initially decided to use the funds. Available evidence suggests that he decided early to allot $5,000 of the appropriation to the navy and to let its officers select one or more limb manufacturers to supply maimed sailors. This, reported Palmer, led Surgeon William Johnson, in charge of the Naval Asylum in Philadelphia, to ask him in early August to furnish limbs for the institution's patients. At the same time, Johnson expressed a wish that all army and navy beneficiaries of the act would be supplied with Palmer limbs.[3]

Palmer proposed Johnson's idea to Hammond and to Surgeon William Whelan, chief of the navy's Bureau of Medicine and Surgery, on August 11, 1862. Palmer hoped that more money would be available for limbs—that "the small appropriation . . . might become the nucleus of a National fund which would confer incalculable blessing on an army of gallant men." He also believed that all parties would be best served if a single maker were selected to furnish all the limbs paid for by the current appropriation, because "to *divide* so small a sum between different Inventors would afford each but an inconsiderable amount, hence the limbs could not be afforded at a price for which they might be made in large numbers." Confident that his devices would be judged superior to others, Palmer added, "As efforts may be made to secure the Government patronage by many incompetent persons, *I would respectfully suggest the propriety of your calling a meeting of all applicants to compare specimens of limbs and prices.*" Adding to Palmer's confidence was his having supplied the U.S. Soldiers' Home with artificial limbs for the past decade. To demonstrate his good faith, Palmer offered to supply twenty-five amputees with limbs at no charge. With his letter to Hammond, the politically astute Palmer included a note of support from Rev. Bellows of the Sanitary Commission, which had supported Hammond's candidacy for the office of surgeon general.[4]

If Hammond had to worry about spending only $15,000—enough for just one hundred Palmer legs at the usual price—devoting a great deal of thought to the matter would hardly have been worthwhile. Perhaps Palmer's letter convinced him that additional funds were likely to be made available and that the matter thus required more attention. In any event, Hammond began assembling his panel of physicians the day after Palmer wrote to him. The current modest appropriation, in fact, was only the beginning of something much larger. Congress would appropriate $66,000 and $45,000 specifically for artificial limbs for the fiscal years ending on June 30 of 1864 and 1865, respectively. Furthermore, additional funds for limbs were obtained from the general appropriation for the medical department for at least the fiscal year ending on June 30, 1864. Given the total number of limbs supplied by the government during the war, the amount it expended on the devices by April 1865 probably exceeded $300,000. Palmer, for one, had good reason to be optimistic about the board's findings, for most of its members had endorsed his products.[5]

The board met at least five times, with Valentine Mott serving as president and Richard Satterlee as secretary. J. Mason Warren could not attend but submitted some thoughts in writing, and Joseph Pancoast did not participate at all because of ill health. At the first session, the panelists reviewed models and the proposed prices from various makers and, unable to come to a decision, invited all limb makers known to them to appear in person with their proposals a week later. Ten such manufacturers did so: Douglas Bly, John S. Drake, Theodore F. Engelbrecht, Henry A. Gildea, E. D. Hudson, Benjamin W. Jewett, Dieterick W. Kolbe, A. A. Marks, B. Frank Palmer, and William Selpho. Three makers—Engelbrecht, Hudson, and Selpho—even brought amputees wearing their limbs to demonstrate how easily and naturally they could move about. The proposed prices ranged from $3 to $15 for a peg leg and from $35 to $90 for an articulated leg. Artificial arms varied more widely in price—from $25 to $135—largely depending on whether the limb ended in a hook or a functional hand with articulated fingers.[6]

Board member Samuel Gross "strongly advocated" peg legs because of their "better adaptation to the wants of the private soldier" but was outvoted by his colleagues, every one of whom favored "supplying each man with the more elegant and costly, but far less durable, [articulated] limb." Thus, at the board's third meeting on September 3, the members settled on "the names of five manufacturers of artificial limbs, who all things considered, they deemed the best, and most reliable, looking to the object of the government." They were Bly, Hudson, Jewett, Palmer, and Selpho for articulated legs. The board did not recommend any peg legs or select manufacturers to provide artificial arms. The lowest proposed price for a leg among the selected makers was $50 from Jewett, with the other makers asking $75 or $90. The board advised that qualified recipients be allowed $50 toward the purchase of an artificial leg and $25 toward the purchase of an artificial arm; recipients would have to pay the difference between the government allowance and the price charged by the manufacturer.[7]

Members of the board met twice with Hammond in September, before a final report was submitted, so the surgeon general knew the direction of—and possibly influenced—the group's deliberations. It is likely he knew by mid-September that Jewett's legs had been judged acceptable and were offered for the lowest price. Perhaps the enormous casualty figures from the September 17 Battle of Antietam—the bloodiest day of the war—spurred Hammond to take quick action, for on September 28, he directed Acting Assistant Surgeon Charles Henry Nichols, in charge of St. Elizabeth Hospital in Washington, D.C., to provide space in the institution so that Jewett could make artificial limbs for the army patients there.[8]

Before finalizing its report, the board sought the opinions of absentee member J. Mason Warren and of Samuel Gross, who had attended only the first two meetings; these views were received shortly after the board submitted the report to Hammond on October 9 and were forwarded to the surgeon general. Warren, writing from Boston, concurred with the recommendations of September 3 whereas Gross did not.[9] Gross's reasoning was compelling:

> My colleagues, I perceive, recommend that the government should appropriate to each mutilated soldier requiring an artificial leg, the sum of fifty dollars, at the same time they present the names of four manufacturers who will not supply the article for less than seventy-five. Thus each soldier, employing these manufacturers, would be compelled to add twenty-five dollars out of his own pocket to enable him to secure a limb. . . . The question may well be asked, How is the poor fellow to obtain the additional sum required to make the purchase? If he cannot command it from his own savings he must either beg it, or do without a leg. But this is not all. In order to enable him to obtain a suitable substitute, he must not only visit the manufacturer but remain sometime near him, thus subjecting him to very considerable additional expense. The sum, therefore, is entirely too small; instead of fifty dollars it should be at least seventy five or eighty. This would not be too much even supposing that every soldier employed Mr. Jewett, who offers his limbs at fifty dollars.[10]

Gross recalled that B. Frank. Palmer had, at the board's second meeting, offered to supply legs at $50 rather than $75 each. He had consequently obtained a written pledge from Palmer to supply 300 legs for the entire appropriation of $15,000. "This is *but half the lowest price I have ever received—is half the amount I am now receiving* from the Government Institution—'Soldiers Home'—in Washington—and is *much below the prime cost,*" Palmer pointed out. "I tender this proposition," he concluded, using imaginative accounting, "as a contribution of $15,000."[11]

Gross, like Palmer, believed it best to award all the business to a single firm. In light of Palmer's proposal, said Gross, "[Palmer] & Mr. Jewett stand on the same ground as it respects the price of their limbs, & the only question, in my mind, is whether they are equal in point of beauty & usefulness. From a careful inspection of them, I do not myself believe that there is any material difference in these particulars. The fact is the limb of Jewett is merely a modification of that of Palmer, & may, for aught I know, wear quite as well & as long." Thus, Gross concluded, the contract should be awarded to the company that could be compelled to repair the limbs at little or no cost for a year and that had well-placed branch offices to limit how far recipients would have to travel to be fitted with a limb. Had Palmer learned of this communication, he would probably have been pleased that Gross recognized Jewett's leg as a copy of his own and disconcerted that the good doctor, who had endorsed his products, could now detect no difference in quality between the two and favored supplying peg legs to the program's beneficiaries.[12]

Once Hammond received the board's final report of October 9 and Gross's dissenting opinion, he took additional quick action. Starting in mid-October, he began to order medical directors in various parts of the country to each designate a hospital to receive amputees for the fitting of artificial limbs. Surgeon William S. King in Philadelphia selected Haddington Hospital, standing at a "pleasant rural location a little way out of the city." Because Hammond took Palmer's offer—300 legs for $15,000— to mean that Palmer would accept $50 each for a smaller number of limbs, he ordered King to make arrangements to have Palmer furnish Haddington Hospital on the latter terms. Hammond determined that no other approved manufacturer would receive more than $50, "that being the price demanded by Palmer and Jewett."[13]

On October 20, Palmer wrote excitedly to Hammond that he had seen a letter from Bureau of Medicine and Surgery chief Whelan stating that "the Board convened by the Surgeon General had advised the adoption of Jewett's & Palmer's artificial limbs"; Palmer was unaware that this was true only so far as Gross opining that the board should choose between those two makers. Furious about Jewett's purported violation of his patent, Palmer begged that any dealings with Jewett be suspended until the surgeon general could be fully apprised of Jewett's misbehavior. Palmer, who had been trying to have Jewett arrested, wanted not only to present his case before Hammond but also to face Jewett in Hammond's presence. He had evidently not yet learned that Hammond had already selected Jewett to supply soldiers at St. Elizabeth Hospital; if that news had reached him, he would likely have been even more frantic in his communication to the surgeon general.[14]

Palmer and Hammond met on October 25, with the former bearing two letters of introduction sure to catch Hammond's attention. One was from Samuel Gross, who described Palmer as having "made more limbs than any married man in Christendom" and "deserving of any favor you can bestow upon him in his peculiar line of business." The other was from another Philadelphia physician, John H. B. McClellan, brother of staunch Hammond supporter General George B. McClellan. During the meeting, Palmer evidently described to Hammond his legal actions against not only Jewett, who seems not to have been in attendance, but E. D. Hudson as well, also for purportedly violating his patents; by this time, Palmer had probably learned that the board had recommended Hudson as a supplier. Palmer must have been somewhat placated by having been selected to supply Philadelphia's Haddington Hospital, but he nevertheless pressed Hammond for permission to supply limbs through his office in Boston. His concerns seemed to have little or no effect on Hammond.[15]

William Selpho, having heard nothing official from the surgeon general, wrote Hammond on October 30 for information and to say that he was "justly entitled" to a contract for artificial limbs because, among other reasons, he furnished them "on as favorable terms as any other responsible maker." Hammond, taking this to mean that Selpho would meet the price proposed by Jewett and imposed on Palmer, $50 per leg, directed Surgeon Levi H. Holden in Cincinnati to make arrangements with Selpho to supply legs for patients in that city and Louisville at that price.[16]

Surgeon Charles McDougall in New York City selected Central Park Hospital to receive amputees requiring limbs and was ordered to make arrangements with Hudson. McDougall and Hudson came to an initial agreement before McDougall learned that the maximum government payment would be $50, so the terms had to be revised, with Hudson agreeing to lower his price to that amount.[17]

Hammond directed Assistant Surgeon General Robert Crooke Wood in St. Louis to make arrangements with Selpho and Douglas Bly to supply patients there and to order Surgeon J. B. Porter in Chicago to arrange with either Selpho or Bly to supply that city. Bly, who had asked $90 for a leg with lateral ankle motion and $75 for a leg without that motion, apparently agreed to supply the latter for $50.[18]

Palmer's usual charge for a leg was $150—"from which," Palmer quickly pointed out, "a great abatement has been made in all cases to the poor"— and he was receiving $100 for each leg furnished to the Soldiers' Home. He had been willing all along to "modify [the price] to any extent that may be *possible*" to secure the entire appropriation of $15,000. "I am not disposed," he explained, "to make the necessity of my fellow-creatures, who fall (mutilated) in the noblest struggle in which a people ever engaged, my opportunity of great gain." Yet some of his associates testified in 1860 that Palmer's cost for making a leg was $65 to $75, and Palmer himself placed the cost at about $75. Hudson itemized his own costs to fabricate a leg for a below-knee amputation and arrived at $72.71.[19]

It is curious, then, that Palmer and Hudson agreed to Hammond's terms of $50 per leg for a nonexclusive share of the $15,000 appropriation, because for those two at least, doing so meant providing limbs at a loss if they were being truthful about their costs. Being recognized as a government-approved supplier of limbs to the country's maimed heroes would have considerable promotional value—the advertisements published by the chosen manufacturers proved that—and providing prostheses for less compensation than originally hoped for may have been a small price to pay for the competitive edge gained. There was, after all, still a large pool of civilian customers, and nobody knew where a good working relationship with the government might lead.

Hammond's views on prices may have mirrored those of Surgeon Charles S. Tripler, who served on a board assembled in October 1863 that interviewed various makers of artificial limbs. According to Tripler, "it is evident that the sum paid by the Government for the soldiers affords a profit to the manufacturers; if not, the contract would not have been taken." Furthermore, said Tripler, his board questioned the makers "under oath and ascertained that they make but one quality of limbs & that the price paid for a leg ($50.00) yielded a profit of nearly one hundred per ct." Hammond knew how eager the manufacturers were for government patronage and how intensely they competed with each other. Palmer, for one, was beside himself at the prospect of Jewett getting any of the government business and was willing to go to great lengths to prevent him from becoming the sole supplier. Thus, the surgeon general's early assignment of low-bidder Jewett to Washington's St. Elizabeth Hospital may have been calculated, in part, to show the other manufacturers that

price was a paramount consideration. Hammond's heavy-handed imposition of the $50 price on Palmer, Hudson, Bly, and Selpho and their ultimate
acceptance of that rate—a third less than what each originally proposed—
suggest that Hammond, like Tripler, believed that even $50 per leg would
provide the makers with a healthy profit and that he was correct.[20]

Hammond considered the arrangements with limb manufacturers not
to be contracts per se. After Surgeon McDougall sent him a copy of "articles of agreement" drawn up by E. D. Hudson, the approved supplier for
New York, Hammond said that such a document was "entirely superflu-
ous" and that Hudson should send to his office a model leg whose features
and quality he would match with every limb supplied to the program's
beneficiaries. Hammond later told another surgeon that "no contracts
have been entered upon with manufacturers of artificial limbs" but rather
that the makers were to be paid upon the recommendation of the board
that had examined and adopted certain patterns. Yet when Hammond
decided to discontinue business with one manufacturer, he referred to
the contract not being renewed, and Surgeon Tripler also referred to the
arrangements as contracts.[21]

The program, as initially implemented, called for eligible soldiers and
sailors—the program did not entitle commissioned officers to a limb—to
be admitted to one of the designated hospitals, where they would be fitted
for limbs provided by the maker assigned to that facility. Manufacturers
would be paid $50 per leg directly by the government. The surgeon gen-
eral did not indicate specifically whether soldiers could pay a maker an
additional amount for a better grade of limb than that furnished for $50,
but his assumption seems to have been that because Jewett and Palmer
were to supply their best (or only) models for that price, so should any
other approved maker.[22]

Palmer had an office in his assigned city of Philadelphia, and Hudson
was based in his assigned city of New York, but the other assignments for
manufacturers made little geographic sense. Jewett, assigned to Washington, D.C., was based in New Hampshire. Bly had offices in New York
City, Rochester (New York), and Cincinnati, yet was assigned to St. Louis
and was a candidate for Chicago. Selpho, based in New York City, was
assigned to Cincinnati and Louisville and was a candidate for Chicago.
In terms of a current presence in the cities where army hospitals served
as centers for amputees, Palmer was well ahead of his rivals; he had offices not only in Philadelphia and New York City, but also in Boston,
Cincinnati, Chicago, St. Louis, New Orleans, and San Francisco. Hudson
was allowed to fit patients at either his New York office or at the city's

Central Park Hospital, and a similar arrangement was probably made for Palmer in Philadelphia. For other locations, army surgeons or agents for the manufacturers probably took careful measurements that were sent to the home offices, and patients would have to wait in or return to the hospital for their limb to be delivered.[23]

On October 18, 1862, the *American Medical Times* published an account of the board's recommendations that was wrong on numerous counts. Not only did it fail to identify all the board members, it omitted Jewett as an approved manufacturer and said instead that Darwin DeForrest Douglass—who had not submitted a proposal or appeared before the board—had been selected as a supplier. Furthermore, it said that soldiers were free to choose among the selected makers and that if a supplier's price exceeded the allowance of $50 for a leg and $25 for an arm, the recipient must make up the difference himself. Where the *American Medical Times* got this information is unknown. The announcement, reprinted in periodicals throughout the country, had some important consequences. First, it confused the limb manufacturers who had appeared before the board, because none of them had yet heard officially about any decisions that the board or surgeon general had made. Second, it introduced to the public and to limb manufacturers the notion of limb recipients' having some freedom of choice in prostheses. Third, it induced manufacturers who had not appeared before the board to request that their products be considered for government approval.[24]

A. A. Marks was disappointed at being omitted from the makers listed in the *American Medical Times* notice. "As some of them are of such small note," he wrote to Hammond, "I wish to know if I am rejected." Marks continued: "I . . . had every reason to believe that my very *low prices* [$50 per leg, or $40 each 'if contracting for all'], in connection with my very *long* standing in the profession would certainly entitle me to a reasonable share at least of the government patronage in this lightley [*sic*] paid branch of a noble charity from our overburdened and benevolent government."[25]

D. DeForrest Douglass saw the original notice and its reprintings in other periodicals and reported that the news of his being named an approved supplier had prompted soldiers to apply to him for limbs. Several such limbs, he said, were currently being made, and he wished to know why he had not received official notification of his appointment. Upon being informed that he had not been selected after all, he wrote again, saying that he had, on the basis of the notice, advertised his selection as a government supplier—in *Scientific American*, for example—and had amputees appealing to him for assistance because they wanted his model over all others. Must those amputees, he asked, "who by the strongest possible testimony, by practical demonstrations, and by a thorough examination of the different legs; are convinced in favor of mine; be compelled to procure the others?"[26] Hammond, who by this time had heard enough from Douglass, instructed a subordinate to name for Douglass the eminent members of the board that recommended the various limbs and to continue the firm response: "From the opinion of such a Board there can be no appeal, and this Board has not recommended your limbs as worthy of the patronage of the Surgeon General. As the Surgeon General, and not a person incompetent to judge, as every soldier must be more or less, has been designated by Congress to choose the proper limb . . . the only accounts paid at this Office will be for limbs ordered by the Surgeon General or his duly authorized agent. Should any Soldiers, deprived of one or both of their legs, apply to you as you have stated, you will serve the purposes of humanity by referring them to Surgeon McDougall, USA, Medical Director New York City."[27]

Douglass was not the only maker upset about the lack of choice on the part of amputees; Palmer voiced the same complaint. "I am prepared to prove that many soldiers have been *compelled* to accept an inferior imitation, (a counterfeit,) of my Patent, *against their will*," said Palmer, "and there are at this moment several soldiers in this city who positively refused to accept legs of other construction, and came to me prepared to pay for their limbs *out of their own small means*."[28]

Appeals arrived at the surgeon general's office from manufacturers who had not originally been considered by the board. Mason Matlack, a Philadelphia-based manufacturer who produced the metallic skeleton legs formerly made by Yerger and Ord, stated that the notices "have said nothing of other manufacturers who make quite as good and better legs than some that have been named. . . . There is now several of the wounded soldiers now in this city who want [the metallic leg] but are told by Palmer that they will have to pay for it themselves whereas if they get thare leg of him the government will pay one half the cost." "All I ask," he concluded, "is if the government is a goin to furnish legs to the soldiers is that they will have the privilige of selecting for themselves if so I should respt ask you in case they should come to me whether the government is responsible for any of the cost or not." George B. Jewett, maker of the Salem leg, had not known that proposals were being considered by the board and presented letters from three members of that board—Samuel Gross, Valentine Mott, and J. Mason Warren—asking Hammond to give the Salem leg a thorough examination. John Fravel of St. Louis had also been unaware of the board and submitted letters, including one from the Western Sanitary Commission, in support of his artificial limbs. Jewett and Fravel were given permission to submit models for examination. Whether a similar invitation was extended to Matlack has not been determined, although Matlack's limb was evaluated by a subsequent board of physicians.[29]

A number of procedural questions arose during the first few months of the program's operation. Hammond informed correspondents, for example, that the congressional appropriation applied to military men who had lost a limb in any war, not just the current conflict, and that the loss need not have occurred as a consequence of combat. Hammond also ruled that amputees who had obtained an artificial limb on their own could not be reimbursed by the government. One former soldier who asked for such consideration had lost a leg at the first Battle of Bull Run and had an artificial limb paid for privately by former Secretary of War Simon Cameron. The veteran, aware of the congressional appropriation, submitted that he had "a claim on said fund from his misfortune at Bull Run, and his having a wife and three little ones entirely dependent on him for support" and therefore asked Hammond "to direct the usual sum to be paid . . . from said artificial limb fund."[30]

On Christmas Day 1862, Douglas Bly requested rulings from the surgeon general on two important points. First, he wished to know whether he was limited to supplying soldiers only through the St. Louis army hospital designated for amputees. Could he also furnish his limbs to any beneficiaries who desired them, regardless of geographic location? Second, although the government payment of $50 applied to his leg without lateral ankle movement, he wondered whether a beneficiary outside of St. Louis could pay an additional fee out of pocket to receive his more expensive ball-and-socket model with lateral ankle movement. That Bly believed he had such permission, at least at St. Louis, was clear in his pamphlets: "[The surgeon general] determined to furnish each soldier who should lose a leg with my Army and Navy Leg [without lateral ankle movement], or one of the others . . . at the same price [$50], and allow those who are able to pay the difference between these and my Anatomical Leg [with lateral ankle movement], to do so, and receive that instead." An answer to Bly's first question—about supplying beneficiaries outside of St. Louis—was to come in a circular released a few days later. Because no direct reply to the second question has been found, it is not known whether Bly ever had authorization at any location to receive payment from soldiers over the $50 paid any approved maker by the government.[31]

Bly, his ball-and-socket leg, and his extra charges were, in fact, particular targets of Palmer as he described his dissatisfaction with how
the limbs program was being operated. While he had been supplying
limbs at a loss for $50 each, said Palmer, "several counterfeiters of my
Patents have been furnishing their *shabby imitations* at the same price;
and one individual [Bly] has been supplying a thing (with 'lateral motion'
in it) which Surgeon-General Hammond has assured me is an *'absurdity.'*
This man has been charging the *soldier* $50 for the 'absurdity,' and the
Government $50 for the *stick* on which it turns." Palmer continued, "Had
a suitable arrangement been made when it should have been [to have
Palmer receive the entire $15,000 appropriation], I could have been pre-
pared to supply the whole demand." Palmer did approve of one aspect of
the program: the decision to supply articulated limbs only. "The Board
rendered a service to *humanity* in yielding to the argument against the
'peg,' and ruled *it* out," he said. "This was indeed a triumph for the soldier."
Palmer's opinions notwithstanding, the effort to supply limbs was getting
off to a slow but sure start.[32]

Program records suggest that the issuing of limbs started in October
1862, with Palmer supplying five of the six legs that month. The *New
York Times*, however, reported that the first government limbs were
furnished—they would have been made by Jewett—for patients at St.
Elizabeth Hospital: "Yesterday [December 9, 1862], for the first time, artificial legs were distributed among the soldiers who have lost their pedal
extremities in the service of their country. . . . The soldiers were much
pleased with the new aids to locomotion, and many amusing scenes occurred among them while trying on their artificial legs. The first individual who tried one was lustily cheered by his companions as he paraded
through the wards of the hospital. All the patients will be supplied in the
course of a few days." Although Jewett, with his early assignment to St.
Elizabeth, should have gotten a jump on the other approved makers, he
was not the busiest in 1862. Of the thirty-eight legs furnished that year,
Jewett accounted for only six; Palmer provided fifteen, Hudson ten, Bly
three, and Selpho one.[33]

The year 1862 ended with a substantial enhancement to the government's plan to supply limbs. A circular dated December 31 described
the new policy: "Hereafter soldiers entitled to artificial limbs, and not
in one of the U.S. Hospitals established for their reception, may, upon
presenting proof to any of the following duly appointed Medical Directors, receive from them an order for the same. . . . These orders may
be given, as desired in each individual case, upon any of the following

manufacturers: Palmer, Selpho, Bly, Hudson, or Jewett, and the price of the limb furnished by these dealers on such orders is not to exceed fifty dollars." The named medical directors were in Boston, New York City, Philadelphia, Baltimore, Washington, D.C., Cincinnati, Louisville, St. Louis, Chicago, and New Orleans.[34]

Thus, soldiers and sailors who were not in one of the designated hospitals could select from the approved makers, although that choice still seemed denied to amputees admitted to those institutions. Artificial arms were not yet available, but that situation would change quickly in the new year as the limbs program gained momentum. The program's growth would lead to the inclusion of additional limb makers, a higher level of service to beneficiaries, and more questions about procedures. It would also be marked by serious allegations of misbehavior by some of the manufacturers.

4

Good and Serviceable Limbs

The duty of the government to the soldiers who have been
maimed or who have fallen in its defence has not been neglected. Much care has been taken, by precautions and practical tests, to secure for the former the most durable, useful, and
comfortable artificial limbs.

—Edwin M. Stanton, Annual Report
of the Secretary of War, 1866

The groundwork established by Surgeon General Hammond provided
a firm basis for the growth of a robust limbs program. Now that
soldiers and sailors who were not in designated hospitals had the freedom
to select their own limb manufacturer, for example, Hammond quickly
added yet another choice, at least for recipients in the Chicago area. In early
January 1863, the surgeon general received a group of endorsements of the
Wilcox patent leg made by Charles Stafford of Chicago. Among them was
a recommendation by Robert Laughlin Rea, M.D., of Rush Medical College, who opined that "for the class of Western patients needing artificial
limbs, especially those performing manual labor, I regard Mr. Stafford's
leg superior to any in use." On February 17, Hammond authorized Surgeon
J. B. Porter in Chicago to obtain Stafford's leg for those military amputees
who desired it, the price allowed not to exceed that paid for other approved
legs ($50). Only one additional leg manufacturer would be newly approved
by the surgeon general before the end of the war.[1]

One of the most glaring weaknesses of the early program was the lack
of approved artificial arms and hands. The original board of physicians
that met in 1862 examined a number of upper-extremity prostheses but
recommended none. Hammond took a step toward correcting the situation in December 1862 by instructing Surgeon McDougall in New York
to "select five soldiers who have suffered amputation of the arm, three

below the elbow and two above and cause them to be fitted by Mr. Selpho with artificial arm and hand." McDougall was to allow sufficient time to judge the value of the limbs and report back to Hammond. The 1862 board had heard manufacturers' presentations, examined devices, and witnessed limbs being worn by amputees who were hand-picked by the makers; certainly having McDougall test Selpho's limbs in new patients would provide a less biased and more practical assessment. It appears that Hammond approved Selpho's arm, for amputations below the elbow, before March 1863 and allowed a payment of $50 each, twice what the 1862 board recommended paying for an arm.[2]

The next models of artificial arms to receive serious consideration were those of Henry A. Gildea of Philadelphia, who had presented an artificial hand to the 1862 board. Gildea sent Hammond a description of his arms in April 1863 and received an invitation to submit models the same month. On May 14, Hammond approved Gildea's models—"in many respects the best yet offered," the surgeon general thought—for both above- and below-elbow amputations at $50 each. Medical directors were charged with deciding "in the individual cases on the propriety or impropriety of furnishing the limb, such decision being based on the probable utility of the limb to the wearer." Hammond asked Gildea to submit drawings and instructions for recipients to measure themselves for an arm; these were to be sent to the various medical directors and given to applicants desiring a Gildea arm.[3]

Hammond's quick decision, evidently made without the benefit of a panel, may have been prompted by his April 23 decision to discontinue further business with William Selpho for charging soldiers "over and above the amount authorized by Govt for artificial legs." Selpho acknowledged the act but begged for leniency, claiming that he had "never received any notice from the medical director further than stating that the government allowed $50 and I naturally concluded that I might charge for extras." Included with Selpho's appeal was a note from John Henry Puleston, military agent for Pennsylvania, who stated that Selpho had "the names of soldiers who have paid extra for some extra work to two other limb makers, & I believe he really did not know he was violating the spirit of his contract, so long as he charged the Govt only the price agreed upon." Selpho's son Edwin, in a separate letter, took the blame and explained that he had acted "without my fathers knowledge, because at that time a severe domestic affliction had overtaken us in the death of my mother, and in consequence of which my father was unable to attend to business." Edwin stated that he was unaware that he was violating the agreement.[4]

Hammond replied that the elder Selpho had previously stated that he would furnish legs on terms as favorable as those of any other responsible maker. As he had done previously when imposing the $50 price on Selpho, Hammond misunderstood or manipulated the manufacturer's meaning, which was simply that he offered competitive prices in regular business. Hammond also pointed to Selpho's acknowledgment of his assignment on the same terms as Palmer's and Jewett's, but there is no evidence to contradict Selpho's assertion that he was told nothing about the terms beyond the $50 government payment per leg. "Thus," concluded Hammond, "there can be no doubt that you understood the terms of your arrangement." Hammond, although evidently unmoved by the explanation of William and Edwin Selpho, still had to deal with the suggestion that other makers were assessing charges to limb recipients. That warranted further investigation and would not be the only indication that other makers were acting improperly.[5]

Sensing that more than one maker of artificial arms would be needed and spurred by an inquiry from Palmer, Hammond called for a board of army surgeons—civilian physicians were omitted from panels from this point forward—to assemble in Philadelphia on June 22, 1863, to examine whatever models of arms might be presented. Palmer claimed to have been inundated with requests for his artificial arm since the discontinuation of the government's business with Selpho and, for soldiers, was willing to accept $75 to $100 per arm, a considerable discount from his usual price of $150. Thinking that the allowance was still $25 rather than the current $50 paid for a Gildea arm, Palmer considered "the *offer* of such a contemptible thing [a $25 limb] to the *soldier*, as an act scarcely less reprehensible than the act of the rebel in shooting off his natural limb." According to Palmer, many soldiers, "not being willing to have the inferior ones made by Mr. Gildea, and others, on any terms," were willing to pay whatever amount the government would not cover for a Palmer arm. He therefore asked that such an arrangement be allowed, as was supposedly being done for Bly and his ball-and-socket leg.[6]

The June 22 panel was dissolved, apparently without submitting recommendations, and another panel—composed of Surgeons Robert Murray, John Campbell, and Andrew Kingsbury Smith—was ordered to meet in Philadelphia on October 14. Upon the recommendations of that panel, Selpho's model for below-elbow amputations and Marvin Lincoln's for above-elbow amputations were approved on December 12, 1863, for a price not to exceed $50. Palmer's arm, said the panel, surpassed all others "for beauty of appearance and symmetry of shape as well as ingenuity of mechanism," but its "close imitation of every joint" seemed to have no "practical advantages except for the sake of appearance," especially when Selpho's arm could perform the same movements and be purchased for much less. Thus, in accordance with the panel's recommendation, soldiers who wanted "the more expensive arm of Palmer" were allowed $50 towards its purchase—provided that a medical director could "satisfy himself that the transaction has been carried out in good faith"—and would have to pay Palmer an additional $50 out of pocket. Palmer and Lincoln came to an agreement whereby arms from both makers were available through Palmer's offices, and Palmer even advertised the availability of the Lincoln model for beneficiaries who selected it as the free government model. For Palmer, who deprecated any devices but his own and referred to other government-approved arms as "sticks and clutches," cooperating with former partner Lincoln and withholding comments about the quality of that maker's arms no doubt tested his restraint. Selpho's reapproval as a supplier evidently signaled his reinstatement as a manufacturer in good standing, perhaps because his previous misdeed of charging more than the government allowance now seemed no different from what Palmer was being allowed to do.[7]

Late 1863 also marked an important change in Washington, which apparently did little to affect the momentum of the Union limbs program: the replacement of Surgeon General Hammond with Surgeon Joseph K. Barnes. Hammond, whose appointment and personality had rankled many career army surgeons and Secretary of War Edwin Stanton, was effectively removed from office when Stanton ordered him out of Washington on an inspection tour in late summer 1863. Barnes was named acting surgeon general in September 1863. A court martial heavily influenced by Stanton convicted Hammond of flimsy charges, and he was officially dismissed from the service in August 1864; Barnes was formally appointed surgeon general at that time.[8]

Yet another panel—composed of Surgeons Richard Satterlee, Charles McDougall, and Bennett Augustine Clements—convened in New York City starting on July 11, 1864, and met nearly daily until August 8. It "minutely examined" fifteen models of artificial legs from fourteen makers and nine models of artificial arms from eight makers. Its recommendations led to the reapproval on August 17 of the artificial arms of Lincoln and Selpho for above- and below-elbow amputations, respectively. Lincoln's and Kolbe's arms for below-elbow amputations were also approved as was Gildea's device for amputations at the wrist. The board concluded that a government payment beyond $50 was "not necessary to secure a good & serviceable arm," but Palmer's arm, even though it was not pre-sented to the panel, remained available for beneficiaries willing to pay $50 out of pocket. The board also expressed a favorable opinion of E. D. Hudson's apparatus for resection of the elbow joint. Selpho's artificial leg, originally approved in November 1862, before business with that maker was discontinued, was reapproved and joined those of Bly, Hudson, B. W. Jewett, and Palmer. The Stafford leg, which had been supplied through the medical director in Chicago, was now made generally available to any beneficiary desiring it. Along with the August approvals came an increase to $75 in the government allowance for legs, necessitated by increases in the cost to manufacturers of materials and labor.[9]

The deliberations of Satterlee, McDougall, and Clements demonstrate the care with which the various devices were considered. The arms, for example, of Hudson and of Kimball and Lawrence for above-elbow am-putations and of Gildea and of Kimball and Lawrence for below-elbow amputations were judged as "good, but adapted only for purposes of dress, delicate use, & remedying deformity, and therefore not well suited for the use of the majority of soldiers." Three devices for above-elbow am-putations were judged not to be good and serviceable: Gildea's because of inability to flex the thumb and fingers and to keep the elbow flexed, A. A. Marks's because of excessive weight and inability to keep the elbow flexed, and Increase M. Grenell's because of an insufficiently perfected and tested mechanism.[10]

The availability of numerous models gave the panel the freedom to elevate its standards and be fairly selective. Thus, although Gildea's de-vice for amputation at the wrist was approved, his arms for above- and below-elbow amputations, which Hammond had considered the best only fifteen months before, were displaced by other devices. Gildea had not been complacent, for he had been improving his artificial hand, at least, by "strengthening parts hitherto supposed sufficiently strong." His experience, he said, had enabled him "to provide better for the rough and careless persons on whom limbs have been fitted than any person could have known by theory."[11]

The board's evaluation of legs was equally discerning. In addition to the models that ended up being approved, the board also recognized those of D. DeForrest Douglass and Marks as good and serviceable, although it was not unanimous in so classifying them and concluded that more time was needed to prove their worth in actual use. Eight models failed to meet the "good and serviceable" criterion. The joints of the Salem leg were too nar-row, and the limb seemed to lack sufficient strength, while the leg made by

Phylander Daniels had defective joints and exhibited "rude construction." The metallic legs of James W. Weston (Theodore F. Engelbrecht's patent) and of I. M. Grenell (an undetermined design) were too heavy and noisy and had too much play in the ankle joint. Joshua Monroe's design was impressive, but its rawhide construction had not been adequately tested. Insufficient testing was also a limitation of the vulcanized rubber leg of Kimball and Lawrence, whose construction was "complicated & delicate." The board declined to consider limbs presented by J. Miller and by Miller and Wells because of "uncertainty as to the ownership & responsibility for them, and of disagreement among the parties."[12]

Boards convened more often now, sometimes to evaluate the products of just one company. Soon after Small and McMillen of Cleveland submitted models of artificial legs for inspection in late November 1864, a panel of surgeons met in Cincinnati to examine them, and its favorable report led to Barnes adding the company on December 20 as the last approved leg supplier of the war. Another board met several times to evaluate Yerger's metallic leg as made by Mason Matlack of Philadelphia and was favorably impressed. Matlack was invited to submit the limb to yet another board "in order that it may be tested in competition with other models." That later board did not approve Matlack's leg.[13]

In January 1865, Barnes approved the artificial arms of I. M. Grenell, even though the board examining them several months before had concluded that they had not been sufficiently refined and tested. As was allowed with Palmer's arm, Grenell was authorized to charge recipients more than the $50 the government would pay—an additional $15 and $30 for limbs made for below- and above-elbow amputations, respectively. It is unclear whether the approval of Grenell was the result of a new panel's recommendations.[14]

The last board before the war's end—composed of Surgeons James Simons, Henry Stewart Hewitt, and B. A. Clements—met from March 15 to May 5, 1865, and was charged with testing "each model as far as practicable before recommending its adoption by actual use upon patients in Hosp." It evaluated legs from twenty-six makers and arms from sixteen, and its recommendations resulted in the list of approved suppliers being supplemented on May 13, 1865, by several other makers: Richard Clement, Marks, and the Salem Leg Company (George B. Jewett) for artificial legs; John Condell and the National Leg and Arm Company for artificial arms; and Hudson and Kolbe for apparatus for resection. The circular showing all the approved devices listed them in order of quality as determined by the board; Bly's ball-and-socket leg, for example, was the top-rated leg, and Marks's was the lowest. Soldiers were responsible for paying the portion of the listed manufacturer's price that exceeded the government allowance of $75 for a leg and $50 for an arm or an apparatus for resection. The devices priced higher than the government allowance were Bly's ball-and-socket leg ($120) and the arms of John Condell ($150), I. M. Grenell ($75), and the National Leg and Arm Company ($80). Marks, who asked $65 per leg, was the only maker whose price was less than the government allowance. Palmer's arm, which was not submitted for evaluation, no longer appeared on lists of approved devices. Manufacturers approved in 1866 included the American Arm and Leg Company, Monroe and Gardiner, and Hiram A. Kimball for artificial legs and Kimball for artificial arms.[15]

The original procedures established by Hammond were refined throughout the war. The requirement that an amputee admitted to a designated hospital be furnished only by the manufacturer assigned to that institution appears to have been dropped by March 1863. During that month, Douglas Bly, one of two manufacturers assigned in November 1862 to supply St. Louis, informed Hammond that he was "preparing stock and materials" and was within a month of "opening a Manufactory of Artificial Legs in St. Louis, Mo., in accordance with your first instructions." The surgeon general replied tersely with what must have been surprising news: "Your order to furnish artificial legs at St. Louis stands revoked at your own expense, and you will be considered on the same footing there as the other manufacturers." Hammond's action suggests that patients in the hospitals previously designated for amputees were now free to select their own limb manufacturer from among those previously approved and that he had neglected to inform Bly, and perhaps other manufacturers, of his decision.[16]

To make the furnishing of limbs more accommodating to beneficiaries, the program allowed a soldier or sailor applying for a device at the office of a medical director to examine manufacturer-provided models then and there. Upon selecting one, he could be given free transportation to a designated city for the taking of measurements and free lodging there in an army hospital while waiting for the limb to be made and shipped back; these benefits were offered even to men who had been discharged from the service. In some instances, a beneficiary was provided with detailed instructions on how to measure his stump for a prosthesis, and the finished limb was shipped directly to him. Artificial limbs furnished to beneficiaries were inspected by designated surgeons to ensure that the devices were of a quality at least equal to that of models supplied by the manufacturers. By late 1864, recipients of limbs were required to wear them for three days before inspection so that they would not go home with an ill-fitting device.[17]

The surgeon general's office found B. Frank. Palmer to be a common source of inquiries regarding procedures. In April 1863, for example, he asked if it would not be proper for the surgeon general to pay the 3 percent ad valorem tax imposed on manufacturers by the revenue act of June 1, 1862. Palmer thought he should not have to pay it himself because he had proposed his price before September 1, 1862, when the tax began to be levied. Hammond was "not prepared to refund the U.S. tax on artificial limbs" and saw no way he could do so. The tax continued in effect until July 1866, when Congress granted an exemption for crutches and artificial limbs, eyes, and teeth.[18]

In late 1863, Palmer sought permission to sell artificial limbs to Confederate prisoners of war. Secretary of War Stanton saw no objection and approved of Palmer not acting on his own but rather "submitting the question . . . as a course proper to be pursued by loyal and patriotic men." Because some of the prisoners were exchanged before their limbs were completed, Palmer asked whether the devices could be shipped south. "When the prisoners have been delivered beyond our lines," he was told, "the same rules will apply then to the furnishing of artificial limbs as to any other article of trade." Trade with the South was generally prohibited, and it has not been determined whether the limbs in question were ever delivered.[19]

Palmer publicized Stanton's permission to supply Confederate soldiers in promotional material for his newly formed American Artificial Limb Company, for which stock was being sold and a healthy return projected. To some, this aspect of Palmer's business was unseemly. "It is very clear," said a California newspaper sarcastically, "that the patriotic and charitable gentlemen who take stock in this company will be heartily in favor of the vigorous and prolonged prosecution of the war" and that such persons would agree that "all who are likely to cut off the demand for wooden legs, are intolerable nuisances, and should be put down by the strong arm of the government." A similar sentiment appeared in a North Carolina newspaper. Palmer probably saw the prisoners not only as a current pool of customers but also as a source of testimonials for the postwar period when the South would be virgin territory for enterprising limb manufacturers.[20]

In May 1864, Surgeon Charles Tripler suggested to Acting Surgeon General Barnes that the approved limb manufacturers be prodded to allow commissioned officers—who were not designated as beneficiaries of the congressional appropriation—to purchase devices at the same price paid by the government. "I know that very many of the officers who have lost limbs are in limited and even straitened circumstances," said Tripler, "& that they cannot afford to pay the price demanded by the limb manufacturers." Tripler, who was convinced that the makers were reaping a handsome profit even at the prices paid by the government, continued: "The price demanded from officers is from $125.00 to $175.00. This appears to me to be exorbitant & I hope some means may be found to induce the manufacturers to reduce the price." Barnes's response has not been determined, and manufacturers' literature does not suggest that officers were charged less than the usual civilian prices. Commissioned officers continued to be excluded as beneficiaries until 1868, when Congress approved supplying limbs to officers up to the rank of army captain or navy lieutenant. The benefit was extended to all officers in 1870.[21]

Allegations of overcharging and other misbehavior by manufacturers must have been particularly troubling to Hammond and Barnes. William Selpho, punished for overcharging, had alluded to similar acts by other makers, and Hammond evidently asked him for details. Selpho named one soldier "who said he paid Palmer's agent in Boston $50 besides the govt order" and another whom he understood to have been charged $50 extra for a Hudson leg.[22]

Surgeon Tripler informed Acting Surgeon General Barnes in June 1864 of the case of Private Absalom A. Overman of Azalia, Indiana, who had applied for a Palmer leg, which was delivered from Palmer's manufactory in Philadelphia to Marsh, Corliss & Co., the maker's agent in Cincinnati. "I am one of the unfortunate boys that lost a leg at Vicksburg," wrote Overman to Governor Oliver Morton of Indiana, "and have made application for a leg." Overman stated that the agent had informed him that he would have to come to Cincinnati to receive the leg and that the charge for freight and fitting would be $10. That charge, said Overman, plus the "cost of going after it will make it cost me as much as though the government had no hand in it." The complaint made its way to Tripler, who thought that Palmer should not be charging anything above what was paid by the government, called the Overman incident "not the first case of complaints of this precise nature" and asked the medical director in Indianapolis for "any facts in your possession going to show that 'extras' are charged to soldiers for limbs on Government orders." Tripler went on in a later communication to say that "The government contract is for the *best limb*, yet there is reason to believe that the manufacturers sometimes exact additional payment from mutilated soldiers." To Barnes, Tripler provided a blunt assessment: "There seems to be no doubt that Marsh,

Corliss & Co. have been guilty of this extortion in Overman's case—& if in that, probably in others." Tripler said he would stop sending orders to the agent until Barnes's instructions were received.[23]

Palmer's Cincinnati agent, in fact, was the subject of other allegations similar to that of Overman's. "Many complaints have arisen," wrote amputee Nicholas Fisher of the 37th Ohio Infantry, "on account of the impositions practiced on the mutilated soldiers by the agent of this place for Palmer's Artificial Limbs." Not only were limb recipients being charged a $10 fitting fee, "the soldier has to pay from four to five Dollars for the transportation of the limb when it is forwarded to him." It appears that Tripler also informed Barnes of overcharging by Douglas Bly, to which the acting surgeon general replied that "Dr. Bly should furnish his best article" for the $50 paid by the government and added that "the means that you have taken in regard to the extortion that seems to have been practiced are approved."[24]

The actions taken in these cases have not been determined, but misconduct by limb makers seems not to have been rare. In some cases, reported Barnes shortly after the war, manufacturers "guaranteeing to supply upon government order, at stated prices, limbs fully equal to those submitted to the boards, have furnished an inferior article or have extorted from the soldier an extra payment for some fancied or nominal improvement." Barnes continued, saying that "in all such cases coming to the knowledge of this department measures have been taken to protect the soldier and punish the criminal party, by requiring the defective limb to be replaced, or the overcharge reimbursed, under penalty of entire withdrawal of government orders."[25]

By April 1865, at least seven manufacturers had been approved to supply artificial legs and five to supply arms, with other suppliers approved after the war. An official report in May 1866 shows the program gaining momentum in 1863 and peaking in 1865, with a total of about 3,800 legs and 2,200 arms being supplied by May 1866 at a cost of almost $360,000 (appendix B). The number of limbs provided to sailors was small—fourteen according to the surgeon general and seventy-one according to the secretary of the navy. In July 1866, the surgeon general estimated that only a thousand or so limbs remained to be supplied. Indeed, by then, the issuance of devices had fallen off sharply. The total number of legs, arms, and apparatus for resection furnished from May 1866 to May 1867 was only 614, just over a sixth of the 3,540 devices furnished in 1865. Thus, in light of the expected delays in supplying an artificial limb—completing the paperwork, waiting for the swelling of the stump to subside, allowing time for the device to be made—the program seems to have been fairly efficient in making prostheses available quickly to those who desired them.[26]

More than half of the artificial legs furnished by May 1866 were supplied by Palmer and Bly, with another 35 percent coming from the other manufacturers approved in 1862—Hudson, B. W. Jewett, and Selpho. Selpho was hurt badly by having his agreement revoked by Hammond in 1863. Not being an approved leg supplier for more than two years in the middle of the war meant that he ended up supplying only about 5 percent of all legs by May 1866, and his total barely surpassed that of the Salem Leg Company, which became a supplier in May 1865.[27]

Marvin Lincoln manufactured almost half of the artificial arms supplied by the program by May 1866. The next most commonly supplied arm was from I. M. Grenell, who made about 18 percent of the devices—this despite his approval not occurring until January 1865 and recipients having to pay him up to $30 over the government allowance. For all his bluster about soldiers clamoring for his arm at any cost, Palmer supplied less than 3 percent of the arms furnished through the program. The need for beneficiaries to pay Palmer $50 over the government allowance may have contributed to his poor showing.[28]

Gauging recipients' satisfaction with the devices provided through the program is difficult at best because no reliable surveys of that variable exist. Palmer claimed to have sent a questionnaire in 1868 to every war amputee he could identify who had received an artificial leg. He selected a representative sample of 400 from the 1,500 to 2,000 responses received and found that, among recipients of a Palmer leg, 90 percent were satisfied; the corresponding figure for recipients of other legs was 3 percent. Since Palmer supplied 30 percent of the program's legs, his results suggest that only 29 percent of leg recipients were satisfied. In light of the fact that Palmer conducted and reported the survey, his findings must be viewed with caution. Barnes acknowledged that not all recipients had "useful and well-fitting limbs." Too often, he said, "the urgency of the applicant or the interest of the manufacturer have acted injuriously in adapting limbs before stumps had entirely healed, or the enlargement resulting from inflammation had subsided, and reopening of wounds, or shrinking of stumps, with consequent inability to wear the limb provided by the government, have resulted."[29]

The percentage of amputees who received devices through the program is unknown, and any estimate would require some fairly broad assumptions. If Union amputation statistics are accurate as to number and survival (they probably underestimate the number), if all amputees underwent only one amputation and received only one prosthesis (not the case), if 6 percent of amputees were officers (a crude estimate) and thus ineligible for the program, and if the roughly 10,000 amputations unlikely to require or unable to accommodate a prosthesis (those beyond the wrist or ankle or at the shoulder or hip) are disregarded, then about 6,400 men were candidates for an artificial leg and 5,500 for an artificial arm. If these denominators are used with the numbers of limbs issued by May 1867 (4,109 legs and 2,452 arms), then 64 percent of eligible leg amputees and 45 percent of eligible arm amputees had received a device. These would be impressive figures by any standard, given the lack of a preexisting program and the huge number of casualties generated by the war.[30]

The wartime limbs program, however ambitious about quality and service, was limited in what it could do for any one beneficiary. "But one limb will be supplied by the Government to each cripple," said one limb manufacturer, "and that must be kept in repair by the owner, and when worn out replaced at his own expense." Furthermore, not all debilitating injuries could be ameliorated by an artificial limb, so Surgeon General Barnes recommended in 1866 that, if the congressional appropriation were to continue, the applicant should receive "the present money value [of a limb] in lieu of an order from a manufacturer." This arrangement, said Barnes, "would include those cases in which, from the nature of the injury and operation, no limb or (surgical) appliance can be advantageously adopted, by extending to them the same allowance now made to their more fortunate fellow-sufferers." These concerns were addressed in 1870 when legislation authorized previous recipients of an artificial limb or resection apparatus to receive a replacement every five years or money commutation in place of the device. The same money commutation was authorized for soldiers who had lost a limb but whose injury did not allow the use of an artificial limb.[31]

The Union limbs program was started de novo with an appropriation so modest that it would pay for only a hundred Palmer limbs at their usual price. A combination of factors—organized and dedicated administrators within the medical department, continued and more generous funding, and an already growing limbs industry that was eager for additional business—helped to develop the effort into one that by May 1867 supplied devices to more than 6,700 military men who had suffered amputation or resection of a limb. Although not all recipients were satisfied with their prostheses, the program was a remarkable logistical accomplishment and an important milestone in the government's commitment to care for its wounded soldiers and sailors.[32]

5

An Act of Esteem and Gratitude

> You must have surmised that the combined effect of the butch-
> ery of war & the surgeon's art must have made many a maimed
> man hobble on crutches or dangle an empty sleeve by his side
> in these C.S. of America. It is even so.
> —William A. Carrington, letter to James Marion Sims, 1864

Excited conversation and oratory resounded through Richmond's African Church on the evening of January 22, 1864. A few days earlier, a committee had drafted a constitution for an organization to supply prostheses to military men who had lost a limb fighting for Southern independence. And now, the public was gathered to officially launch the association and hear Confederate States senators Albert G. Brown of Mississippi and Gustavus A. Henry of Tennessee, a grandson of Patrick Henry, urge all Southerners to lend their support.[1]

The organization was the brainchild of the Reverend Charles K. Marshall of Mississippi, who was noted for his efforts to relieve the suffering of sick or wounded Confederate soldiers. Marshall—so the story goes—had recently visited a hospital and observed a soldier examining an artificial limb. The price of the Richmond-made prosthesis, $300 in Confederate currency, was well beyond the means of most soldiers, and the clergyman instantly hit upon the idea of raising money to provide the devices at no charge to army and navy amputees. Although the idea of such assistance had arisen in the Confederate Congress in 1863, no action had been taken. Thus, the need for forming a benevolent association to supply limbs was the subject of handbills and newspaper notices that Marshall published in Richmond on January 12, 1864. That appeal was quickly followed by the constitution-drafting meeting.[2]

The "enthusiastic and earnest crowd" assembled at the African Church learned that the new organization had been named the Association for the Relief of Maimed Soldiers (ARMS). The ARMS constitution was read and approved, and officers were elected, pending their willingness to accept the positions. They included Marshall as president, Richmond banker William H. Macfarland as treasurer, a corresponding secretary, a recording secretary, and a board of directors. The twelve vice presidents, each representing a different Southern or border state, were Confederate legislators or other prominent figures. By the end of the meeting, ARMS had become the only Confederacy-wide program of its sort and was off to an encouraging start, with nearly $20,000 of contributions in hand.[3]

Although a private organization, ARMS was strongly supported from the start by the Confederate Army Medical Department. Among the nine directors, for example, were Surgeon General Samuel Preston Moore, Surgeon James Brown McCaw, and Surgeon Charles Bell Gibson; McCaw and Gibson each directed an army hospital in Richmond and taught at the city's Medical College of Virginia. The most important army appointee was Surgeon William Allen Carrington—medical director for hospitals in Richmond and chief administrator of all general hospitals in Virginia—who served as corresponding secretary for the new organization. The office of corresponding secretary supposedly carried little responsibility, yet Carrington ended up running ARMS's day-to-day operations and using his army connections, privileges, and prestige to further the organization's aims. Marshall had secured Carrington's assistance early, and the latter was seeking out limb manufacturers at least two days before the ARMS constitution was drafted.[4]

Finding those manufacturers was a challenge. Before the war, persons in the nonindustrial South who needed artificial limbs generally got them from the North, where "mechanical pursuits"—and the accidents attending them—were more common. Among the firms that Carrington initially contacted were G. W. Wells and Brother of Charlottesville, Virginia, and J. E. Hanger and Brother of Staunton, Virginia. Little is known of George W. Wells's origins as a limb maker, although his firm had fit ninety-seven legs by early 1864, including prostheses for Generals Richard Stoddart Ewell and John Bell Hood, and had orders pending for about a hundred more. James E. Hanger was one of two Southerners to lose a leg as a result of the June 1861 Battle of Philippi, Virginia (now West Virginia), and later claimed to be the Civil War's first amputee. The young Hanger—he was only eighteen when wounded—returned home from his brief stint with the army, in which he had never officially enrolled, and successfully fashioned his own workable artificial limb "chiefly of barrel staves." Word of his accomplishment spread and appeared in local newspapers, and Hanger started making limbs for other amputees. By the time Carrington contacted him, Hanger held the only two Confederate patents for artificial limbs and also had orders from waiting customers.[5]

Carrington's search went beyond those with established limb-making experience. He wrote to H. M. Smith of Richmond, who was recognized, said Carrington, "as one of our most ingenious manufacturers" but evidently not known to have ever fashioned an artificial limb. "I will be happy," added Carrington, "to assist you by showing you any of the writings on this subject or to show you such limbs as are in my reach." A similar letter went to a Mr. Gibson, whose handiwork, a "plain stump" made for an amputee, had caught Carrington's eye. "As you are an ingenious man," said Carrington, "and have much experience in the manufacture of instruments and machines, I suggest that you give some thought and attention to this matter of artificial limbs, and see if you cannot devise some cheap, simple, strong, and durable apparatus." Gibson estimated that he could provide peg legs for $55 each if made one or two at a time and for $40 each if manufactured in batches of a hundred or more.[6]

Indeed, to Carrington and the ARMS directors, a simple peg leg seemed sufficient at first. "The Directors think," wrote Carrington to Wells, "that such a leg as you make will not be required by many applicants. A man engaged in agricultural pursuits will be as well suited with a cheap, plain substitute consisting of a good socket (as in your leg) & to this a wooden shaft neatly turned with a ring of iron & a heel of leather or gutta percha." Repairs on such a device, said Carrington, would be less frequent and less costly than on one with movable joints at the knee, ankle, and foot. Wells replied that "very few indeed would be satisfied with the styles of leg suggested" and supported his view by summarizing an informal poll of leg recipients, "all of whom seem to agree that such a leg would be very uncomfortable and far less adapted to their use & comfort than the one we are now manufacturing." Wells did acknowledge that "the leg you propose could be less expensive and more liberally compensate us for our work."[7]

Not himself an expert in artificial limbs, Carrington eagerly sought advice, written information, and specimens of prostheses. He asked Wells about the difficulties in fitting artificial legs, the surgical techniques that produced stumps best suited for the devices, and postsurgical neuralgia. From Rufus R. Rhodes, Confederate commissioner of patents, Carrington sought information about prostheses invented by Southerners. "The [artificial limbs] patents before the war as published in the Patent Office reports are *all* Yankee," Carrington lamented, but he asked Rhodes's assistance in reproducing drawings of them, not only for his own edification, but for that of actual or potential limb makers. Pamphlets or actual specimens of Northern legs—models by Palmer, Bly, and Yerger and Ord, for example— were obtained, some from persons arriving from the United States in flag-of-truce boats. Carrington familiarized himself as best he could with the various Northern designs and concluded that Bly's was probably the best.[8]

One specimen came to be examined by ARMS under most unusual circumstances. During the night of March 2, 1864, a Union cavalry foray toward Richmond led by Colonel Ulric Dahlgren ended disastrously for the Yankees when Confederate troops ambushed the raiders, shot Dahlgren to death, and captured many of his men. On Dahlgren's body were found papers that purportedly indicated that one aim of his mission was to assassinate Confederate president Jefferson Davis and his cabinet. While Richmond and the rest of the South raged over this discovery, Carrington sought another item reported to have been removed from Dahlgren's body: an artificial leg. Dahlgren had obtained it after a foot wound received in July 1863 had forced amputation of his lower leg.[9]

Dahlgren's body and prosthesis were delivered to Richmond separately, and now Carrington asked Secretary of War James Alexander Seddon that the leg be turned over to him. "I am having made many artificial legs for maimed soldiers," said Carrington, "and wish to examine this to see if any improvements can be discovered in the mode of manufacture." Unaware of the exact whereabouts of the limb, Carrington speculated that "the officer who brought the body to the city, no doubt, has the information." Hearing that General Fitzhugh Lee had been involved, Carrington sent a similar letter to that officer and added that he "had seen it [the leg] in the possession of Surg. Chs Bell Gibson (one of the [ARMS] Directors) who informed me that it was only loaned him. If it is considered the private property of some one of his captors, I would be obliged to you for information or his name &c as we would willingly buy it." The leg, Carrington informed Wells on the same day, was a Jewett model, "very handsomely enamelled but it is inferior to Bly's leg." By early May, the leg had found its way to Wells, who made drawings of it at Carrington's request. The prosthesis afterward belonged to various owners—including two Confederate cavalrymen who each wore it to replace his own amputated leg—before being recovered after the war by Dahlgren's father, U.S. Navy admiral John Dahlgren.[10]

Carrington initially knew of no person who could manufacture artificial arms or even seemed knowledgeable about them, so he wrote to renowned surgeon James Marion Sims, a South Carolinian living in Paris. "I consider *you* a Confederate," wrote Carrington, "and as such I request that you procure me as soon as possible & send me specimens of the most approved artificial arms manufactured in England & France; and also if there is any improvement in legs, not known until the last few years, send me a diagram of one showing the improvement." Despite such appeals, including some to Confederate sympathizers in the United States, the association had "no good model or specimen [of an arm] at our disposal; & the U.S. Patent Office Reports show none that is worthy of a copy." Carrington had a Palmer pamphlet containing "a diagram of his arm with a description in full. It is not very convenient and I think not very simple. I have made a diagram of an English arm, which I found with a friend. It is broken and almost repaired out of all its original features."[11]

Carrington also solicited assessments of artificial limbs from credible sources. In a note written to Wells and forwarded to Carrington, General Ewell praised his Wells-made prosthesis as "altogether superior to any I had before been able to obtain. . . . It differs from the others . . . in not causing injury to my stump. I am able with it to walk a short distance without even the aid of a stick, and with one, I can get along pretty well, which was never the case before, though one of the legs previously used by me was made in Paris—though not made to my measure. Dr. [Hunter Holmes] McGuire Medical Director assures me he considers the legs made by you superior to the celebrated Palmer legs." Ewell's physician, Surgeon Francis Woodson Hancock, noted that the general had used two other Virginia-made legs—one, by a Mr. Bundy of Haxall's Mills, which he considered a "very excellent leg, well balanced & light; [but] being about the first made was scarcely strong enough for long continued severe use"; and the other, made by William Bradley of Manchester, being "very clumsy and entirely too heavy for the General's strength." From what he had seen of Wells's legs, Hancock judged them "very good . . . probably the best."[12]

Other generals had lost a leg, and it was difficult to keep them on duty when artificial legs were so hard to obtain. Thus, Surgeon John Thomson Darby, acting on oral instructions from the secretary of war and surgeon general, had been ordered to Europe in November 1863 to help alleviate the situation. He took with him, according to a newspaper account, "models of the truncated members of a number of Confederate officers" so that artificial limbs could be custom made. The devices "were supplied in sets of two or three each, that, amidst the perils of blockade-running, one at least should reach its destination in safety." Darby, the account continued, took especial care of one leg, "sewing it up in a waterproof casing, that it might survive the chances of being thrown overboard to be rescued from the clutches of Federal chasers." That limb, made by Frederick Gray of London, was meant for General John B. Hood, who had lost a leg at Chickamauga.[13]

Darby returned in April 1864 and received a request from Carrington for information. "I am afraid," remarked Carrington, "that Gray's [Anglesey model] leg has not fulfilled your sanguine expectation as I see from a newspaper sketch that Genl Hood has been on crutches." A crutch, replied Darby, was necessary because Hood's arm, wounded at Gettysburg, was too weak to allow the use of a cane, which would otherwise suffice. As for the Gray leg, Darby opined that "for durability, lightness, strength & freedom of motion at the knee joint . . . [it] surpasses any leg I have seen in the country or Europe." The French designs he had seen were "inferior to the Charlottesville [Wells] limb, first worn by Gen'l H. being fully as heavy and more clumsy."[14]

Carrington also asked to examine General Matthew Calbraith Butler's leg—also a Gray's model obtained by Darby in England—and to hear the general's opinion about it. Butler replied that he would be glad to oblige when he was next in Richmond and added, "Suffice it to say for the present that I have very little inconvenience in walking short distances and ride as well as ever." Carrington sent a similar request to General William S. Walker. A Union surgeon had amputated Walker's leg after the general rode unintentionally into Union lines and was shot in the lower leg and elsewhere after refusing to surrender. While confined, Walker learned that an aunt in New Jersey would supply him with an artificial leg if he could come to New York. His resultant application for a parole was declined, so surgeons at Fort Monroe, where he was hospitalized, made measurements and a plaster cast of his stump and sent them to a Northern maker. According to a Union surgeon, the leg arrived, fit nicely, and allowed the general to walk quite well. Walker was eventually exchanged and answered Carrington's inquiry by saying that he had suffered a serious fall and had consequently not yet begun using his prosthesis. It is unclear whether he was referring to the same leg that he had received while a prisoner; Carrington thought the general used a Hudson leg.[15]

The endorsements received about the Wells leg and the terms the firm offered—$125, $150, and $175 per leg for amputations below, at, and above the knee, respectively—convinced ARMS officials to designate Wells as the association's first supplier of artificial legs on February 10, 1864. Soldiers and sailors, including commissioned officers, who submitted satisfactory proof that they lost a leg while serving the Confederacy would receive an order on Wells for a prosthesis, which would be furnished at no charge. Surgeons James Lawrence Cabell and John Staige Davis, both stationed at Charlottesville, consented to inspect each Wells leg, and if satisfied, endorse the bill to be submitted by Wells to the ARMS treasurer.[16]

Hanger submitted terms, a detailed description of his design, and a sample leg and was approved on March 12, 1864, as ARMS's second leg supplier. His model, made until recently of steel, was a modification of the Palmer pattern. Hanger had recently switched to "very light wood" that was "enveloped with raw hide which strengthens the wood much more than leather or any other material & then painted varnished &c." Surgeons William Hay and John Charles Martin Merillat, stationed at Staunton, agreed to serve as inspectors. Hanger was to receive $150 per leg for below-knee amputations and $200 per leg for at- or above-knee amputations. He thought he could supply ten to fifteen legs per month, or as many as needed as long as he had enough workmen. With two suppliers now available, applicants for an artificial leg could specify which maker—Wells or Hanger—they preferred.[17]

Even if Wells and Hanger operated at full capacity, they could not keep up with the anticipated demand, since Carrington estimated in March 1864 that some nine thousand already wounded men would be applying for an arm or leg, with more than two thousand likely to be maimed in the next campaign. Carrington estimated that the two firms could together produce two hundred legs a month, an inexplicably optimistic figure, given Hanger's and Wells's guesses that they could perhaps furnish fifteen and thirty limbs monthly, respectively. In any event, the ongoing need for manufacturers spurred Carrington to call for assistance in the April 1864 issue of the *Confederate States Medical and Surgical Journal*, which was edited by ARMS board member Surgeon James McCaw. Artificial legs, said Carrington's article, "can be made very easily by any good locksmith, gunsmith, instrument-maker, or ingenious mechanic." Those of Wells and Hanger, he added, combined "lightness, strength and symmetry" and were "worn with comfort and satisfaction by officers and men in the field and in every station of life, civil and military."[18]

One response to the article came in May 1864 from Surgeon Littleton Upshur Mayo, who said he could manufacture a thousand legs—an improvement on Palmer's design—within eighteen to twenty-four months and deliver them in lots of twenty-five or thirty. Mayo, who did not explain how he could carry out his proposal while also fulfilling his duties as an active-duty surgeon, was court-martialed for reasons that are unclear and dismissed from the army in September 1864. Carrington, still hoping that Mayo could assist, informed him in October 1864 that each limb had to be individually fit to the applicant and that large batches could not be produced in predetermined sizes as trusses or shoes were. Another offer to provide limbs was tendered by Christopher H. Summersett, a former

North Carolina infantry lieutenant who had been dismissed from the army for prolonged absence without leave. Now employed at the Confederate navy yard at Wilmington, North Carolina, Summersett had invented "a leg . . . of very simple construction modeled in wood after the human leg" that to Carrington "seemed to be deficient having no joint at the foot & only an axis at the ankle joint with a steel spring acting by pressure." It appears that neither Mayo nor Summersett was awarded a contract.[19]

Other prospects seemed somewhat more promising. Levi Davis of Fluvanna County, Virginia, was making limbs and had more orders than he could handle but evidently had not been in the business long. The 1860 census listed Davis as a wheelwright, and his partner, William B. Hodgson—who lost a leg as a child and wore a Davis prosthesis—referred to himself in 1864 as a merchant. Albert Strasser of Montgomery, Alabama, had invented an artificial limb and started a business, Strasser and Callahan, to produce them. William T. Cole of Columbus, Georgia, was charging $450 to $500 for legs and provided a detailed and impressive description of his product. "My legs so far as I know," he said proudly, "have given perfect satisfaction and I do not think it presumptuous when I say for elegance and durability they are not surpassed by any made in our country." G. W. Spooner, a former Wells employee, proposed to furnish a leg designed by Thomas R. Dolan, who had also worked for Wells. Spooner partnered with R. F. Harris, who had been making gun carriages and grapeshot and canister balls, to form Spooner and Harris in Wells's town of Charlottesville.[20]

"The difficulties of transportation and postal intercourse are such," noted Carrington, "that maimed men cannot, without great suffering and delay, come to Virginia to secure the benefit of the Association." Thus, Carrington thought it particularly important to pursue the Montgomery and Columbus prospects. Among the candidate firms, Cole and Spooner and Harris, reported Carrington, were "extensively engaged in manufacturing the limbs and make legs of suitable properties. The prices they propose, however, are double those hitherto paid by the Association." ARMS expressed an intention of working at least with Cole, Strasser and Callahan, and Spooner and Harris, and contracted with the latter two firms. It appears that Spooner and Harris, which received a contract on January 2, 1865, was the only firm of the three to receive orders from the association.[21]

Notwithstanding the compliments paid to Hanger and Wells in his *Confederate States Medical and Surgical Journal* article, Carrington was not always pleased with the quality of their work. Surgeon Hay reported from Staunton in March 1864 that the Hanger legs he had seen were "very indifferent in fact if they were a fair sample of their work, I think the Association would be throwing its money away to purchase them as the men who have them have been obliged to throw them aside & go back to their pegs." A "much disconcerted" Carrington informed Hanger of this assessment and told him that applicants from Hanger's region of Virginia were asking for a Wells leg. "I relied on you to supply many of the men now applying to me," continued Carrington, "and now tell you this with the request that you let me know where I can see legs of yours in successful operation, and persons to whom you can refer & to whom I can write." Carrington could have cited the example of applicant Leroy Daingerfield—from Bath County, next to Hanger's home county of Augusta—who wanted a Wells leg. Daingerfield and Hanger had each lost a leg on the same day from wounds received at Philippi.[22]

In January 1865, Carrington, who had just seen a limb furnished by Hanger, sent an angry letter to Surgeon Archibald Magill Fauntleroy, who had succeeded Surgeon Hay as a limbs inspector in Staunton: "It is made in workmanship inefficient and *very* inferior to the specimens he [Hanger] deposited with the Association. The color is unsightly the toes are not fastened by hinges as the specimen was, but by wooden pegs which will soon be worn off. The braces to the knee are too straight and not curved to the convexities of the knee. The sole leather thigh box made of leather much too rough and too rough entirely. The color with specimen was near flesh color. I am dissatisfied with the leg and hope you will not pass any more such, as these are a discredit to the Association and will soon be of little use to the men."[23] Fauntleroy replied that, according to Hanger, "the artificial limb [referred to] did not differ initially from the limbs they have furnished during three or four months past. During which time they have used the wooden pegs to secure the toes & the color of which you deprecate." Fauntleroy continued, "I have never seen the pattern deposited with the ARMS and my only standard was the limbs which I have noticed in the possession of soldiers during my service here."[24]

Carrington was more forgiving of apparent faults in Wells's work. ARMS president Charles K. Marshall informed Carrington that "I constantly meet with men with Wells leg with the joint out of order & hinges broken & making so much noise in walking as to annoy the wearers & the way the work is badly done & I think that worth looking into. I hear from others that the poplar they use is liable to split easily." The secretary of war, too, had "been informed that the legs furnished by Wells & Bro. were of such inferior mechanism and make as to be useless." Carrington asked that the Wells limbs be inspected more carefully and told Marshall that Wells "makes the handsomest I have seen & is very anxious to do all he can. He makes all repairs free of charge & I believe makes no more than a bare living by his labours." To Wells, Carrington offered reassurance: "I saw General Ewell last night who spoke in very favorable terms of your leg and expressed a desire to remove the unfavorable impression that existed in the mind of the Sec of War." Carrington gently chided, "You have used badly seasoned wood in some of your limbs from complaints made to me."[25]

As if providing artificial legs was not problematic enough, Surgeon Cabell, limbs inspector at Charlottesville, informed Carrington of something else needed by soldiers who were furnished a prosthesis: a suitable pair of shoes. "Many perhaps a majority of [ARMS] beneficiaries are unable to procure the light shoes which for a time at least are indispensable for the exercise of the new limbs. The heavy shoes issued by the [Quartermaster] Dept are entirely unsuitable until by continual practice the maimed soldier has acquired the power of manipulating the limb with such heavy & stiff appendages. The proper kind of shoes can be bought here: but at a very high price viz about seventy dollars." ARMS agreed to pay for such shoes. Wells worked with one Hezekiah Taylor, whom ARMS initially paid $50 (later $65) per pair for shoes that were "low quartered– lined & bound and made of good material to secure as much flexibility as possible." Hanger found a shoemaker who demanded $100 per pair, which Carrington considered too much. Hanger ended up working with a Mr. Williams, who initially charged $65 per pair but asked for $75 per pair after his contract expired. "We think," said Hanger, "if we succeed in getting a detail for a free negro, who is an elegant workman, that we will be able to furnish them at the same price as heretofore." Carrington asked Lieutenant Colonel Aurelius F. Cone of the Richmond quartermaster depot whether shoes for amputees "could be made here by the Govt work shops & furnished or whether they could be furnished in Charlottesville Va where most of the legs are now made there being large manufactories in Charlottesville who probably have contracts with the C.S." As if to convince Cone of the greater good that might result, Carrington added that ARMS "enables [maimed soldiers] to perform light duty."[26]

Carrington's frustration at not being able to furnish artificial arms seemed near an end when he heard from William Bradley, an agent of the Manchester (Virginia) Cotton Mills. Carrington knew that Bradley had fashioned a disappointing leg for General Ewell, so he was probably pleasantly surprised with what Bradley had recently sent. "It affords me pleasure," Carrington told him in November 1864, "to state that the artificial arm and hand you have made gives me satisfaction. Such I think could be worn by the maimed, be very useful, and prevent their being annoyed by impertinent and curious questions. . . . I request that you manufacture for [ARMS] such an arm as you have furnished me and that you make a proposition for a contract for that purpose, stating terms &c &c. We have no person manufacturing them and many hundreds of applications have been received." The next month, Carrington asked Bradley to make an arm for a lieutenant from a Virginia regiment and to charge the device to ARMS, but no other artificial arms are known to have been ordered by the association.[27]

The objects of ARMS extended beyond the furnishing of artificial limbs to include the provision of "such mechanical compensation of other lost parts of the human body, as may be practicable." Consequently, Carrington was asked whether "an artificial jaw would legitimately come under the object of [ARMS]." According to the inquiry, "the soldier referred to had his lower jaw—all the part connected with his teeth at least—shot away, making a frightful wound, his recovery from which was almost miraculous. He is now nearly well, but he eats & articulates badly. The dentist says a silver jaw may be inserted which will be a great help to him, at a cost of about $400, in present currency. He is a very deserving man, & the main support of a widowed mother." Carrington replied that an artificial jaw did "not come under the objects of the Association; at least, the Directors have so decided at a recent meeting, principally because the labor of supplying legs and arms to the thousands of maimed soldiers seemed at present sufficient in magnitude for their capacity." Carrington recommended seeking donations to help pay for the jaw "in preference to waiting until after the War, as the parts will contract until smaller than in health if this action is deferred." In keeping with the wider goals of ARMS, Carrington asked a European contact to send him some glass eyes if funds were available, but there is no evidence that they were received.[28]

Indeed, merely furnishing legs—arms might have to wait until after the war, thought Carrington—was challenge enough. Wells and Hanger were beset with difficulties almost from the start, and ARMS itself, although blessed with generous contributions when first established, struggled to raise money afterward. Yet ARMS did manage to survive and provide limbs—"not as an act of charity, but esteem, respect and gratitude"—albeit not to the extent that the Union limb program did. How it did so is a story of dedication, personal sacrifice, and resourcefulness in the face of almost overwhelming obstacles.[29]

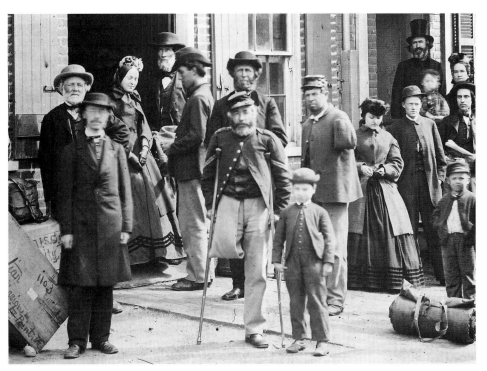

Maimed Union soldiers among a crowd at the office of the U.S. Christian Commission in Washington, D.C. The overall death rate for soldiers undergoing amputation was about 25 percent. Library of Congress (LC-B817-7720).

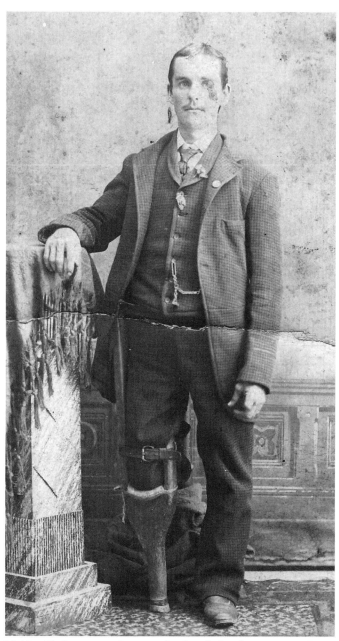

Unidentified man wearing a peg leg for a below-knee amputation. The upright along the outside of the leg attached to a waist strap. Peg legs offered the virtues of simplicity, durability, and economy.

National Museum of Health and Medicine (photograph NCP 4076).

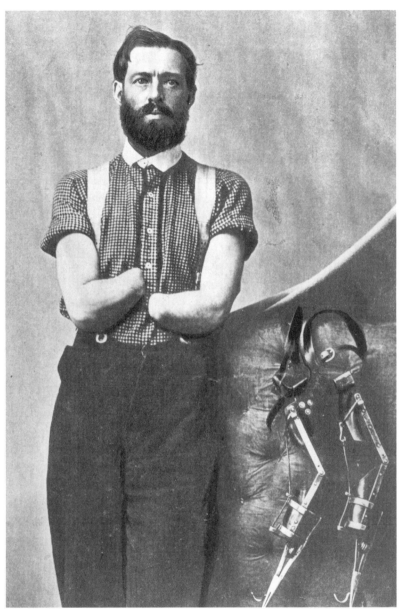

Samuel H. Decker of the Fourth U.S. Artillery, who had both forearms blown off by the premature discharge of his gun on October 8, 1862. He provided himself with artificial limbs that enabled him to write, pick up small objects, carry objects of ordinary weight, and feed and clothe himself. He proved to be an able doorkeeper at the House of Representatives. National Museum of Health and Medicine (photograph SP 205).

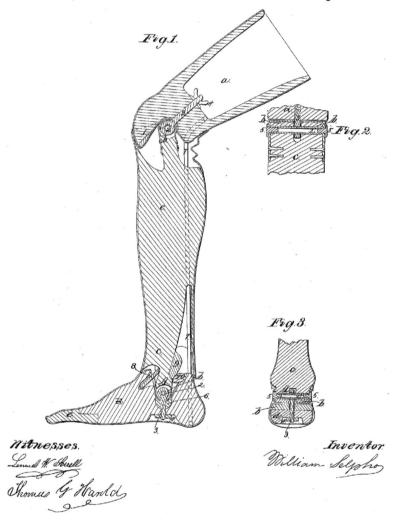

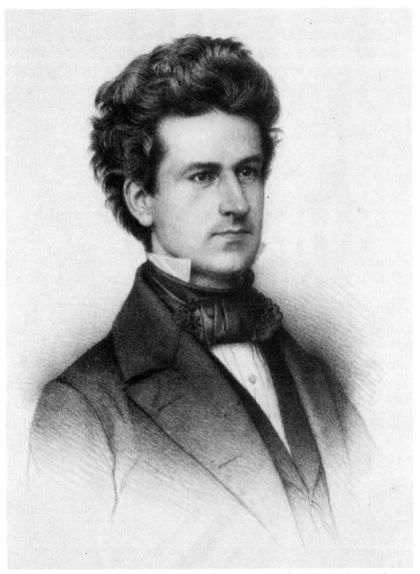

Benjamin Franklin Palmer, a major manufacturer of artificial limbs during the mid-1800s. Palmer, who lost a leg as a child, was granted the first two U.S. patents for artificial limbs. Images from the History of Medicine, National Library of Medicine (image 186149).

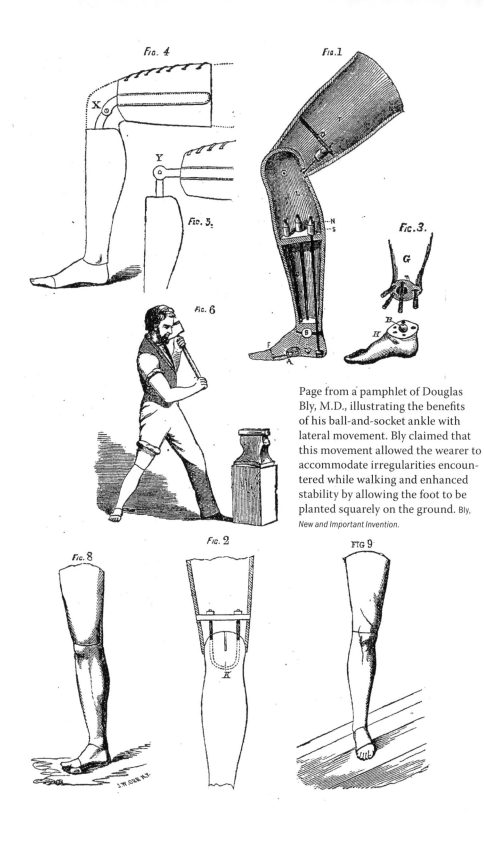

Page from a pamphlet of Douglas Bly, M.D., illustrating the benefits of his ball-and-socket ankle with lateral movement. Bly claimed that this movement allowed the wearer to accommodate irregularities encountered while walking and enhanced stability by allowing the foot to be planted squarely on the ground. Bly, *New and Important Invention.*

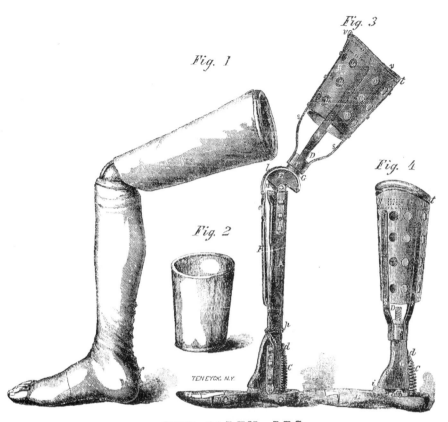

Fig. 1

Fig. 2

Fig. 3

Fig. 4

TEN EYCK. N.Y.

THE SALEM LEG.

Illustrations of the Salem leg designed by George B. Jewett. This model differed from most others in having as its primary structure a wooden tibia rather than a hollowed section of willow wood. A leather cover, stitched along the back, was stuffed with hair to give the limb a somewhat natural contour. Jewett, *Salem Leg.*

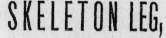

UNITED STATES ORTHOPEDIC INSTITUTE.

M. W. MATLACK,

Late Foreman, and Successor to JOHN F. ORD,

No. 145 North Seventh St., below Race, Philada.,

MANUFACTURER OF

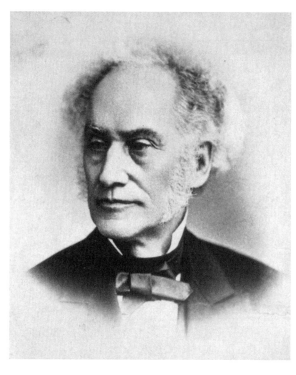

PATENT METALLIC

FOR WHICH

PREMIUMS

BY

SCIENTIFIC

INCLUDING

WORLD'S

SKELETON LEG,

HAVE BEEN

AWARDED

DIFFERENT

ASSOCIATIONS,

THE LONDON

FAIR,

Improved Patent Premium Instruments for Curved Spine, Club Foot, Bow Legs, Knocked Knees, Weak and Sprained Ankles, Ununited Fractures, &c   Also a superior article of Split Crutches.

Hawkes Pr. 717 N. Second St,

Business card of Mason W. Matlack, who made the metallic skeleton leg designed by George W. Yerger. Matlack to Edwin M. Stanton, December 1, 1862, entry 12, Record Group 112, National Archives and Records Administration.

Eminent civilian surgeon Samuel David Gross, who as a member of the first panel to evaluate devices for the Union limbs program advocated supplying soldiers with peg legs rather than articulated models. He also believed that the amount of money that his fellow board members recommended allowing soldiers for the purchase of limbs was inadequate. Images from the History of Medicine, National Library of Medicine (image 178765).

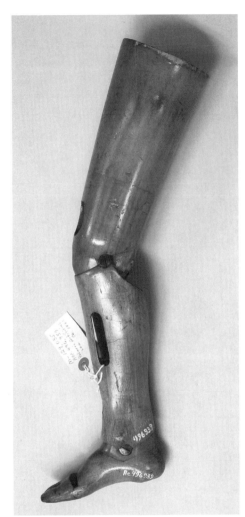

Artificial leg made by B. Frank. Palmer. This specimen, probably fashioned from willow, lacks the usual rawhide covering. Palmer legs were the most commonly supplied by the Union limbs program during the war. Historical Collections, National Museum of Health and Medicine (catalog no. M-129.00035).

Advertisement by E. D. Hudson, M.D., from the January 1863 issue of *Braithwaite's Retrospect of Practical Medicine and Surgery.* Hudson's mention of his commission for the Northern Division refers to his being the only manufacturer assigned in the fall of 1862 to supply the army's Central Park Hospital in New York City. Like many others, this advertisement mentioned prominent physicians as references.

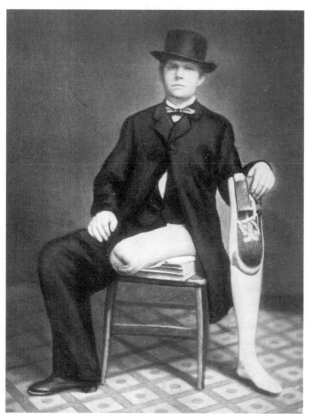

Corporal David D. Cole, 2nd New York Cavalry, who was wounded at Amelia Court House, Virginia, on April 7, 1865, and underwent amputation at the knee on August 1, 1865. Cole was sent to New York in late 1865 to have an artificial limb fitted by E. D. Hudson, M.D. National Museum of Health and Medicine (photograph SP 199).

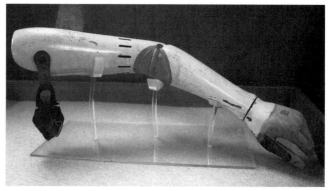

Artificial arm made by Marvin Lincoln for amputation above the elbow. Objects could be held between the fixed fingers and spring-loaded thumb. Courtesy of the National Museum of Civil War Medicine.

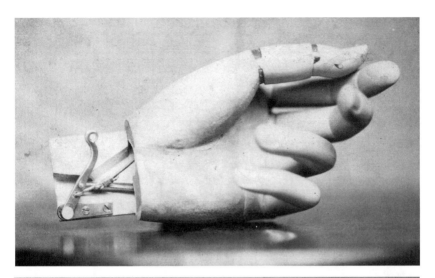

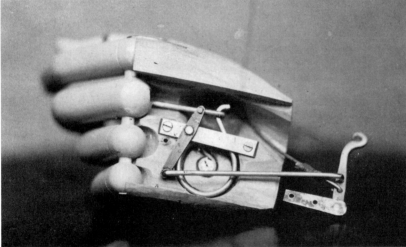

Two views of an artificial hand made by Henry A. Gildea of Philadelphia. The interior mechanism includes a spring, lever, and connecting rod that operate the fingers and a cord that operates the thumb. National Museum of Health and Medicine (photograph CP 1629 [*top*] and CP 1630 [*bottom*]); Gildea to William A. Hammond, July 31, 1863, entry 12, Record Group 112, National Archives and Records Administration.

Corporal John H. Jaycox, 143rd New York Infantry, who underwent removal (resection) of 5½ inches of the head and shaft of the humerus. He was fitted with an apparatus for resection by E. D. Hudson, M.D., which was intended to restore function to the arm. National Museum of Health and Medicine (photograph CP 1219).

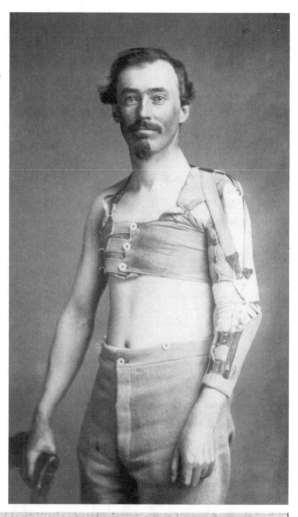

Advertisement by James W. Weston for an artificial leg patented by Theodore Engelbrecht, from the February 21, 1863, issue of *Harper's Weekly*. Although Weston offered a discount to soldiers, he was not an approved supplier from whom soldiers could get a leg at no cost.

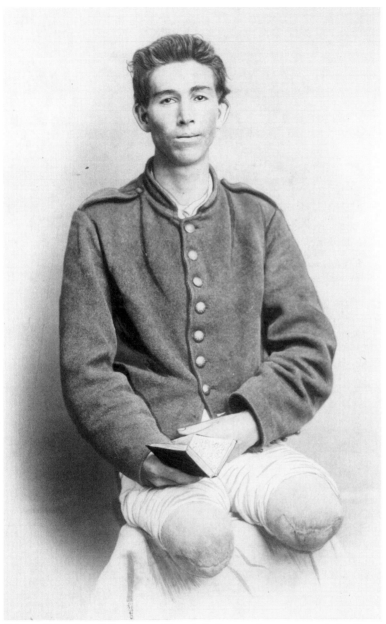

Private Columbus G. Rush, 21st Georgia Infantry, who was wounded at Fort Steadman, Virginia, on March 25, 1865, and had both legs amputated at the thigh by Union surgeons. Rush was fitted in February 1866 with artificial limbs made by E. D. Hudson, M.D. National Museum of Health and Medicine (photograph CP1216, with additional information from photograph SP 132).

James E. Hanger, who
began making artificial
limbs after having
his leg amputated
in 1861 at the age of
eighteen years. In early
1864, the firm of J. E.
Hanger and Brother, of
Staunton, Virginia, was
approved as a limbs
supplier for the Asso-
ciation for the Relief of
Maimed Soldiers. Hanger
Prosthetics and Orthotics.

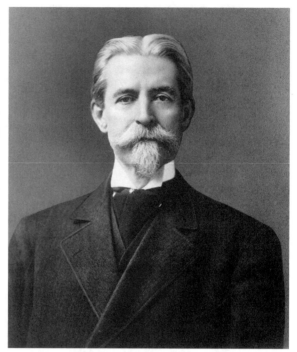

James Lawrence
Cabell, who was a
Confederate surgeon
stationed at Char-
lottesville, Virginia,
and acted as a limbs
inspector for the As-
sociation for the Relief
of Maimed Soldiers.
In 1866 Cabell served
on a board meeting in
Richmond to evaluate
artificial arms and legs.
Images from the History of Medicine, National Library of Medicine
(image 137878).

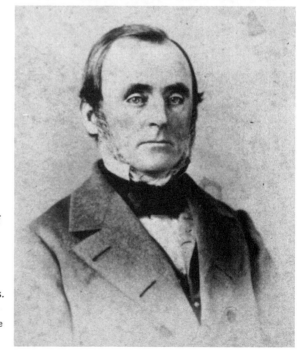

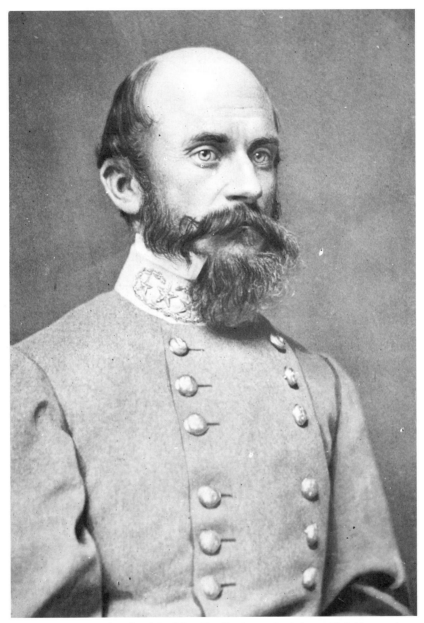

Confederate general Richard Stoddart Ewell, who praised the artificial leg made for him during the war by Wells and Brother of Charlottesville, Virginia. After the war, Ewell provided a testimonial for a leg made by Northern manufacturer Richard Clement. Library of Congress (call no. LC-B813-6583 C).

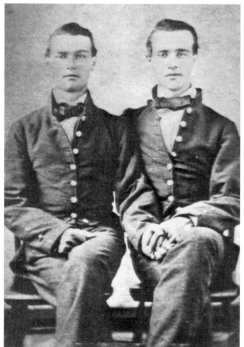

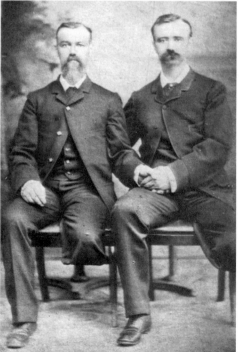

Brothers Levi J. and Henry J. Walker shortly after enlisting in the 13th North Carolina Infantry (*top*) and after the war (*bottom*). Each was wounded in July 1863 and had his left leg amputated. Levi received a leg from the Association for the Relief of Maimed Soldiers, and both received a limb after the war from the state of North Carolina.

Courtesy of the North Carolina Office of Archives and History, Raleigh (photograph N.89.3.25-A for both images); Maxwell, "Two Brothers"; Wegner, *Phantom Pain*, 236–37.

6

MANIFOLD DIFFICULTIES

As is evident the Association is advancing but slowly and by no means in proportion to the requirements of the objects proposed; but considering the absorbing nature of the other duties of most of its officials and the perfect whirlwind of action and the events in which all are involved we can congratulate ourselves that we have organized to set forward prominently the objects of the Association.

> —William A. Carrington, Report of the
> Corresponding Secretary, ARMS, 1864

I dentifying and coming to terms with manufacturers was a vital step but by no means the only difficulty in furnishing Confederate amputees with prostheses. Indeed, the South's artificial-limb makers faced the same obstacles that hindered the Confederacy's other businesses: a scarcity of skilled workers, shortages of vital materials, and ever-increasing prices. Even if firms such as Wells and Brother and Hanger and Brother could overcome such problems, ARMS still had to raise enough money to pay them.[1]

Confederate conscription acts in effect shortly after ARMS was formed declared that all able-bodied white men between the ages of seventeen and fifty years were subject to military service. Certain exemptions were allowed, and men with special skills could be detailed from the army to work for industries deemed vital to the war effort. Army commanders complained that the detail system was abused and seriously compromised the strength of their fighting forces, and the military situation in 1864 and 1865 dictated that details not be too liberally granted. Carrington recognized that detailed conscripts would be vital for the success of ARMS and promised his assistance—details were requested through the secretary of war—in securing them. "You will receive the aide of the

Assoc in securing the details of such men as you require," he assured Wells in February 1864.[2]

By next month, Wells was already asking for help: "The details which should have been renewed the first of this month have not come to hand. ... We are *much* in need of workmen, as we are not able with the present force to furnish more than from twenty eight to thirty legs a month, and you are aware that the number of orders we are receiving daily are largely disproportionate to that. .... We know of no men, outside the army, whose service we could engage." Cognizant that the conscription bureaucracy and the increasing need for troops made obtaining details far from automatic, Carrington advised Wells to "advertise in several of the Richmond papers for such workmen as you require. I suppose gunsmiths or men experienced in manufacturing clocks, watches ... or other complex machinery are the kind you want. .... They should be men not liable to military duty on account of being foreigners or for disability or being of non-conscript age." Hanger was in a similar predicament. The very existence of the firm of Spooner and Harris depended on obtaining detail status for "first class mechanic" and "able bodied conscript" G. W. Spooner and for limb-designer Thomas R. Dolan to run the shop. Detailed conscripts not only provided labor, they freed supervisory personnel to perform important tasks. "No details have come yet & consequently we are completely locked up here," wrote Wells. "We are out of materiel of some kinds that cannot be bought here. You see the disadvantage we labor under in not having details so that we can go off to procure materiel. Please give it your earliest attention & have the details forwarded as soon as possible."[3]

The manufacture of artificial limbs was evidently not considered important enough for the generous granting of details. Carrington got around this obstacle by requesting details in the name of the medical department and sending them to the general hospital in Staunton or Charlottesville. Once there, the ARMS inspectors, who were also surgeons in the hospitals, assigned the details to the limb maker in town. John M. Hanger—the brother in Hanger and Brother—escaped military service until October 1864, when he was enrolled in the 5th Virginia Infantry. "Since my brother left, I find it very difficult to keep the work going on as before," lamented James Hanger, "for I am obliged to be out of the shop a considerable portion of my time & being deprived of his assistance the great & principle [*sic*] inducement to carry on the shop viz the improvement of my work, is taken from me." Yet Carrington managed in mid-November to have John detailed and ordered him to report to Surgeon Fauntleroy, ARMS inspector in Staunton, who assigned him to Hanger and Brother for the duration of the firm's contract.[4]

Those assigned to Wells could even board at the general hospital in Charlottesville. Surgeon Cabell, hospital director there and ARMS inspector, wrote to Carrington for instructions: "Presuming that as heretofore men so assigned will be paid exclusively by the contractors and not be entitled to any pay or rations from the government I desire to know what price shall be charged for their board. Heretofore I have charged two dollars & a half a day to a detailed man on duty with Wells & Bro but the actual cost of the ration used exceeds three dollars. On the other hand the very low charges of the contractors make it imprudent for them to pay heavy wages to their employees."[5]

Carrington's attempts to secure details were not always successful, possibly because he sometimes had to request that conscripts be assigned directly to a limb maker rather than to the medical department in his own jurisdiction of Virginia. He asked, for example, that William Engleheart of the 2nd Alabama Cavalry be detailed to Strasser and Callahan in Montgomery, Alabama. His request, forwarded to Secretary of War James A. Seddon with the approval of Surgeon General Moore, was returned with Seddon's terse reply: "I can not detail a soldier for such work."[6]

Shortages of materials needed to fabricate artificial limbs were noticeable but not critical when the contracts for Wells and Hanger were awarded. When Carrington asked Wells in March 1864 to specify "the *tools & materials* most necessary for manufacturing artificial limbs . . . that cannot be found without difficulty in this country," Wells specified "brass wire, sheep skins & gum elastic" to be among the "few articles which we find any difficulty in procuring." When Hanger submitted a specimen leg to ARMS in February 1864, he explained that the painting was "deficient in appearance only on account of the difficulty in getting the proper material." Carrington reacted quickly by writing to Paris, France, in March 1864 to ask J. Marion Sims to assist "in procuring *files*, brass wire for springs—gutta-percha or india-rubber, & some of the other constituents of the legs."[7]

By August 1864, the situation had deteriorated considerably, both in the availability of materials and the value of Confederate currency. Citing January 1864 prices for comparison, Wells explained why the contract terms no longer provided a "fair and honest living." Sole leather, for example, had increased from $6 to $12 per pound, and screws had increased from $3 to $25 per gross. "Sheepskins *then* $50.00 to 60.00 per dozen," he said, "*now* $300 & have to search the country for them." Hanger summed up the situation after Carrington complained about the appearance of a Hanger leg: "The cost of the material to finish a limb properly in addition to the present cost of the material of which the legs are made would amount to much more than we get for them after they are made. . . . We think that if the ARMS would increase our pay in the same ratio with the increased value of specie (or depreciation if necessary) that we would be able to finish our legs as you desire. When our contract was made last spring specie was worth only 10 to 20 [dollars in Confederate notes] to 1 [dollar in gold]—now it is worth from 60 to 80 per 1 so that our present pay at present prices of any & everything amounts to almost nothing at all. Material of every kind keeps pace with specie." Hanger was not exaggerating about the rapidly widening gap between a gold dollar and a Confederate one. In Richmond, the price of a gold dollar was $22 in Confederate notes when his contract was made in March 1864. The Richmond price of a gold dollar was $50 when Hanger wrote Carrington in early January 1865 and reached nearly $67 later that month.[8]

In response, ARMS instituted a strategy to provide the limb makers with lower-cost materials. One facet of this plan was to purchase cotton and ship it to England, where the profits from its sale could be used to buy materials at a lower cost there than in the South. For this venture, Carrington solicited the assistance of William C. Bee, the executive officer of a large importing and exporting company in South Carolina. Bee predicted that the assent of the company's board of directors to Carrington's appeal, "worded as it is by the silent and touching appeals presented by our brave and afflicted cripples, every where," was certain. Indeed, Bee eagerly offered to assist in the cotton's purchase, its shipment to Nassau at no charge, its transport to Liverpool, and its sale in England. Purchase of the initial lot of cotton would cost $10,000. "As the funds of the Association are now reduced," Carrington advised ARMS, "I suggest that some of the Directors advance the necessary sums or borrow it on their joint note and send it to Mr Bee immediately for expenditure and shipment of the cotton." The sum was provided by ARMS vice president George A. Trenholm, who was senior partner of an importing and exporting company and had recently succeeded Christopher G. Memminger as Confederate secretary of the treasury. At least eleven bales of cotton were subsequently purchased and shipped to Nassau. The cotton was to be received and sold in England by Fraser, Trenholm and Company, of which George Trenholm was also a senior partner.[9]

Carrington called upon Major James B. Ferguson, Confederate quartermaster agent in Liverpool, to use the proceeds from sale of the cotton to purchase a list of goods and to "send triplicates of the articles by different vessels . . . care of our agents in Nassau" and thence to whatever Southern ports might be open. Carrington's list included two widths of elastic cloth (1,000 yards each), 150 pounds of one-eighth-inch brass wire, 60 boxes of plated shoe eyelets, 200 pounds of Irish glue, 24 hacksaw blades, 3,000 suspender buckles, 500 sheets of copper, and 50 sheets of brass. That these items could be purchased in triplicate—in hopes that one shipment would arrive safely in the South—and still save money for ARMS speaks to their drastically lower prices in England than the Confederacy. ARMS records do not document the arrival of the cotton in Liverpool or the purchase of goods by Ferguson.[10]

Carrington also used his connections to obtain assistance from organizations within the Confederacy. The quartermaster general agreed to provide limb makers with a limited number of rawhides and sheep skins at cost. Railroad officials were asked if they could provide "carspring India rubber old or new, in large pieces or scraps to use in the manufacture of artificial limbs." The Confederate Nitre and Mining Bureau, responsible for obtaining the materials needed to produce gunpowder, agreed to provide iron, steel, white paint, and zinc at cost or contract prices. Carrington was particularly interested in the materials needed to give the limbs an appealing finish. "Please inform me," he wrote Wells, "about what are the ingredients of the paint you use for your legs & in what proportion & what is required to make such paint as I see on Northern legs. I find the white lead, zinc, linseed oil, yellow ochre, vermillion, & scarlet carmine can be procured in Richmond as well as varnish of various kinds." Zinc, said Carrington, "is better than lead [for paint] I am told by parties. A little yellow ochre and vermillion should be added to give a flesh color and the whole ground up with turpentine alone and English white copal put on afterward, when it is perfectly dry." Wells and Hanger benefited from Carrington's efforts by ordering at least rawhides, sheep skins, iron, and steel.[11]

A manufacturers' tax also burdened firms like Wells and Hanger. Hanger appealed to his congressman for an exemption, and Carrington backed him up by informing the legislator, "I will be happy to do anything in my power to effect this object as they are very laborious men who do not more than make a living from this very patriotic and benevolent trade." Carrington told Wells, "I will try & have all the work done for the assn relieved from all taxation. I believe that you should only be taxed on your actual clear profit."[12]

Carrington's interventions on behalf of his manufacturers would mean little if ARMS could not pay them for the limbs. ARMS was formed with the hope that assistance would be offered by the Confederate, state, and municipal governments. Carrington, in fact, considered it "a matter of probability that the Confederate States Congress may consider it the due of each Confederate victim of battle to be provided, at public expense, with the best substitute of his lost member that is known to art." Part of the campaign to garner official government support was to ask the various ARMS contractors to submit samples of their work to put on display in Richmond. "They will be seen by thousands, and by members of the *C.S. Congress,*" Carrington told one maker. Nevertheless, ARMS "was designed to appeal principally to benevolent and patriotic Confederate citizens." Membership in ARMS entailed an annual fee of $10. Three hundred dollars would entitle the donor to a life membership, and $1,000 would make the donor an honorary director of the association.[13]

Early donations ranged from $20 from "a Lady" to $2,500 from George A. Trenholm and $5,000 from E. M. Bruce, another vice president of ARMS. "The contribution that gave more encouragement to the officers of the Association than any received" was $500 from General Robert E. Lee in March 1864. Lee became the association's first honorary director when officers and patients of Richmond's Chimborazo Hospital contributed $1,000 in his name; Lee donated another $200 in December 1864.[14]

Among several other honorary directors was General Nathan Bedford Forrest, in whose name the requisite donation was made by "negroes of the Methodist congregation at Uniontown, Alabama." The donors, wrote Carrington to Forrest, "requested that their subscriptions might be thus appropriated to testify their respect and affection for you as their defender. Allow me to say General, that though not so directly under obligations to you, we do not the less admire the great skill and energy that has been exhibited by you during your long and brilliant career."[15] Forrest, in acknowledging the honor, referred to his part in the alleged massacre of black Union soldiers at Fort Pillow:

> I prize this manifestation on the part of the negro more than I fear the thousand calumnies with which a defeated and vanquished foe are endeavoring to blacken my name. It has been my fortune to have much dealing with the negro since I arrived at manhood, and I have uniformly treated them with kindness and humanity.... Those that heeded not the ridiculous promises of the Yankees, and who still remain with me, fly from his approaching footsteps with the same instincts of fear and danger that they would fly from a leprosy.... Instead of being guilty of the atrocities charged upon me, I have uniformly expressed my sympathies

for the negro. He has been deluded by false promises, and I had much rather make war upon the white man, who has deceived him.[16]

The ARMS vice presidents were evidently selected with the intent that their prestige would aid in obtaining contributions from the various Confederate states. One such person was Vice President Alexander Stephens, who declined to serve as an ARMS vice president because of his pressing responsibilities. Carrington asked that he reconsider: "The office will devolve no duties on you, being honorary as far as you are concerned. The object of the Association in soliciting the use of your name was to secure the influence & prestige of your name *alone*, which, the object being worthy, it was hoped would not be denied." Stephens did not reverse his decision.[17]

ARMS also intended to employ one paid agent per state to solicit contributions from its citizens. Candidates for agency might, Carrington thought, be suggested by state governors, and the agents might themselves employ a limited number of subagents. ARMS succeeded in hiring only two agents, Reverend Julius L. Stirewalt, whose territory was Virginia's Shenandoah Valley, and Reverend Philip P. Neely, who covered North Mississippi and Alabama. Carrington was particularly impressed with Stirewalt, who had "collected $35000 in the Valley of Va from the crushed & oppressed inhabitants" by January 1865. "Your success in raising funds to meet the objects of the Association for relieving maimed soldiers has been most creditable both to yourself and to the people of the valley," Carrington told Stirewalt. "You have shown yourself to be the right man." Stirewalt helped establish local ARMS chapters and so impressed citizens that the proceeds from one branch were donated with the request that he be named an ARMS honorary director.[18]

Neely, on the other hand, encountered skepticism at Columbus, Mississippi. "I have presented the claims of your Association to the people of this place and have been much disappointed with the result," reported Neely to Carrington. "The people are frightened at the late tax law [and are] inclined to hold on to what money they have." They also had doubts, said Neely, that ARMS could actually carry out its aims. Nevertheless, Neely raised nearly $19,000 by January 1865 and earned Carrington's gratitude.[19]

Thinking that appeals to citizens' patriotism and benevolence might not be enough, Carrington wrote to Secretary of War Seddon with an idea. "I desire information," queried Carrington, "whether, if a limited number of capitalists (say four or five) be induced to subscribe the capital for the manufacture of limbs, on a large scale, for maimed soldiers, whether they themselves will be exempted from service." There is no evidence of Seddon approving the suggestion.[20]

ARMS also turned to the various state governments for assistance. The surgeon general of North Carolina, Edward Warren, informed Carrington in October 1864 that his state had ordered materials for three thousand artificial limbs from Europe and would shortly establish a state limbs manufactory. In the meantime, North Carolina would reimburse ARMS for what the organization had spent in furnishing its state's soldiers with artificial limbs. Warren reported to North Carolina governor Zebulon Vance in November 1864 that "a number of our soldiers have been supplied with limbs [by ARMS] at the expense of my department," but by March 1865, ARMS had received neither funds from North Carolina nor a response to Carrington's repeated messages. At that time, Carrington informed Vance that ARMS would continue to supply the state's soldiers with limbs gratis but that the reimbursement agreement was considered terminated. Carrington's October 1864 appeal to Governor Pendleton Murrah of Texas, which was supported by Francis R. Lubbock, the former Texas governor and then aide-de-camp to President Davis, is not known to have produced results. Louisiana donated $10,000 in February 1865. Georgia, South Carolina, Alabama, and Mississippi were also on Carrington's list of potential donors.[21]

Europe seemed a likely source of donations, so Carrington asked quartermaster agent Ferguson, stationed in Liverpool, to see if various Southerners residing in England or France might become ARMS members. Carrington also had his eye on a particular sum of money raised by British subjects sympathetic to the Confederate cause. In October 1864, a bazaar was held in Liverpool to aid the Southern Prisoners' Relief Fund, with the intent that the money raised would purchase extra food and clothing for Confederate soldiers held in Union prison camps. A "committee of English gentlemen," headed by Lord Wharncliffe, president of the Southern Independence Association of London, was formed to administer the bazaar's proceeds, which totaled some £17,000, worth about $170,000 (U.S.) at 1864 exchange rates. Wharncliffe asked Charles Francis Adams, U.S. minister in London, whether the U.S. government would allow an agent to visit the camps and "minister to the comfort of those for whom this fund is intended." Adams forwarded the request to United States secretary of state William H. Seward, who angrily rejected it, remarking that "the sum thus insidiously tendered in the name of humanity" consisted in part "of the profits which its contributors may be justly supposed to have derived from the insurgents by exchanging with them arms and munitions of war for the coveted productions of immoral and enervating slave-labor." The correspondence among Wharncliffe, Adams, and Seward was published and produced the expected indignity in the South.[22]

Carrington saw an opportunity and determined to "make an effort to have some of that English gold so insultingly rejected by Mr. Seward. I will try to induce Lord Wharncliffe to perceive that I will not disdain English gold and that Confederate sufferers are accessible to relief." Carrington wrote Wharncliffe, "You were not allowed any open opportunity to carry out your benevolent intentions but were rebuffed with insult. . . . I request that you will . . . consider the facts & aid us in repairing the savages of war, if the objects [of ARMS] & the mode of attaining it meet your approval." It has not been determined whether any of the requested funds were donated to ARMS.[23]

One expense that ARMS managed to avoid was for the transportation of soldiers to and from the towns where the limb manufacturers were located. Soldiers being transferred on government orders received transportation free of charge from the Quartermaster Department. Thus, Carrington bypassed charges by ordering ARMS beneficiaries transferred from an army hospital near their home to one in Charlottesville or Staunton and then back again. Carrington wanted to see any beneficiary, with his new leg, who might be passing through Richmond, so such soldiers received transfers to a Richmond hospital with instructions to visit Carrington's office. Such transfers, emanating as they did from Medical Director Carrington and involving hospitals in Virginia, were not questioned, yet they probably exceeded the bounds of official propriety, since they involved the operation of a private organization and were hardly military necessities.[24]

An amputee whose application for a limb was approved reported to the limb maker for measurements and returned when notified that the limb was ready for fitting. One way of reducing soldiers' travel and inconvenience, Carrington thought, might be to use a preprinted form to send the limb makers the measurements of a stump instead of having the measurements taken by the makers in person. This would remove the need for the beneficiary to return, or stay in town, until the prosthesis was ready for final adjustments and fitting. "I do not see any difficulty in measures being taken this way," opined Wells, "provided the person that took them knew what he was doing. We should invariably work to the measure sent us." All limb makers knew that stumps shrank and changed in shape as healing progressed. "If they are made to fit the stump new, when the stump heals, the leg will be too large," said Hanger. Thus, Carrington ordered that "no legs should be fitted to men whose stumps are unhealed." The problem with makers relying on measurements taken by someone else was that "all persons who want legs want them long before the stump is old enough to receive them," and the readiness of a stump for a prosthesis was best judged by someone well experienced in fitting the devices.[25]

Carrington also hoped to secure free transportation for ARMS agents. Agents Stirewalt and Neely traveled from town to town soliciting contributions, and their expenses had to be reimbursed by ARMS. Carrington's request for government assistance received a disappointing response from the secretary of war: "I do not see my power to grant this application despite its just claims to my sympathy."[26]

In his pleas for assistance, Carrington consistently exaggerated the accomplishments of ARMS. He told William Bee on October 25, 1864, that he had furnished "nearly four hundred legs to maimed soldiers already" and wrote Texas governor Murrah two days later that "some 500 have been supplied with good artificial legs." The actual number delivered by late October was closer to 270. Carrington was well aware of the difference between orders and deliveries. In an internal ARMS report on October 10, for example, he said that of 499 legs ordered, "224 have been furnished and paid for." In March 1865, he wrote two politicians, "I respectfully represent that the Assn for the RMS through its officers have supplied gratuitously 806 officers sailors & soldiers with artificial limbs," but the actual number supplied was closer to half that and included no sailors. Carrington also told Governor Murrah in October 1864 that ARMS had made "contracts in the States further South [than Virginia], and now four large manufactories are working for us." At the time, contracts had been made only with Wells and Hanger of Virginia, so the overstatement may have reflected a belief that agreements with Cole of Columbus, Georgia—which never materialized—and with Strasser and Callahan of Montgomery, Alabama, were imminent. Perhaps Carrington believed that exaggerations of ARMS's efficiency would give potential donors more confidence that their contributions would produce a tangible benefit.[27]

Despite all the efforts to economize and raise money, ARMS was constantly accruing bills in excess of its revenue. The association invested more than $59,000 in Confederate States bonds in April 1864 and sold them in July 1864 at a loss of almost $11,000. Consequently, ARMS paid the first bill from Wells—$7,925 for fifty-three legs, approved in April 1864—two months late and was able to do so only because of a $5,000 advance from ARMS treasurer William Macfarland. By January 17, 1865, total ARMS revenue was $113,464, but expenditures were $122,958, for a deficit of $9,494. The situation was perhaps partially attributable to the meager participation of the civilian members of the ARMS board of directors. "The Directors," said Carrington, "oppressed by other duties, have not been able to give any attention to this matter, except at their meetings." In fact, a committee composed of Carrington and board members Surgeon General Moore and Surgeon McCaw was appointed to attend to all ARMS business except that handled by a separate finance committee, which was charged with appointing agents and raising funds, tasks in which Carrington was also heavily involved.[28]

Carrington demonstrated his own dedication to the organization not only by his tireless work but by putting up his own money to keep its operations going. One payment, used to help finance the shipment of cotton to England, "was advanced by me to the Assn as the agents who have received subscriptions have not sent them on." In another instance, Carrington reported that "The Treasurer having invested all the funds of the Association in 8 per cent bonds was unable to pay the bill of Mr H Taylor, contractor for furnishing shoes for the beneficiaries of the Assn, and as he needed the money at once to go beyond the mountains to buy leather to make other shoes I advanced him the amount—1850$—in CS new issue notes."[29] Carrington's frustration finally caused him to unburden himself to ARMS president Marshall in February 1865:

> I am afraid that you have gone off & left me with the bag to hold. . . .
> Not being incorporated & giving all the orders for legs I will be held
> responsible by manufacturers for their bills, if the Assn does not protect
> me. I am disposed to think that the other gentlemen associated with
> us in this undertaking are not treating me with justice. I have daily a
> great deal of work to do; to which I have not objected to devote most of
> the hours other officials use for recreation or private objects. And yet
> though the duties assigned me in the constitution should make me less
> responsible than any other officers except the recording secy, I am the
> only one to advance my private means to save the assn from discredit
> & when I make the fact known no officer has offered to share the risk
> with me or attempted to relieve the finances of the assn.[30]

Carrington seemed to have forgotten the early large donations from ARMS vice presidents Bruce and Trenholm, Treasurer Macfarland's advance of $5,000, and Trenholm's donation of $10,000 to fund the purchase of cotton.[31]

Despite his indignation, Carrington continued his efforts on behalf of ARMS. On March 6, 1865, he asked ARMS vice president and Confederate senator Louis T. Wigfall of Texas and politician and lawyer Alexander R. Holladay of Virginia for their help in getting the government to approve four benefits: first, gratis transportation for "all maimed officers soldiers & sailors maimed in the service of the C.S. traveling to manufactories for artificial limbs & back to their homes & posts of duty"; second, the purchase by ARMS "at cost or contract prices of any article that may be needed by the assn or its agents in the manufacture of artificial limbs from any one of the departments of the government that can furnish them"; third, "the exemption or detail of any such of its expert workmen & mechanics as the directors will certify to be indispensable"; and fourth, "the exemption from taxation of the funds of the assn & of all work done for the assn by contractors." A "Bill for the Relief of Maimed Soldiers" (Senate bill 221), containing Carrington's wording almost verbatim, was quickly introduced and passed in both houses of Congress, and President Davis approved the legislation on March 11, 1865.[32]

By granting free transportation, the act removed the need for Carrington's questionable practice of transferring ARMS beneficiaries from hospital to hospital. In regard to the assignment of details, the legislation gave ARMS a priority on par with other activities considered vital to the war effort. It blessed the kinds of arrangements that Carrington had already made privately with the quartermaster and the Nitre and Mining Bureau, and it provided for much-needed tax relief to ARMS and its contractors. Unfortunately, the act came more than a week after Union troops occupied Staunton and Charlottesville—where Hanger and Brother, Wells and Brother, and Spooner and Harris were based—and less than a month before the surrender of the Army of Northern Virginia. The surviving records of ARMS end on March 31, 1865, with a notation about the February account of Hanger and Brother.[33]

From its inception in January 1864 to March 9, 1865, ARMS issued 768 orders for legs. Through late April 1864, Wells received all orders, accounting for about 180. Of the subsequent orders, about 350 went to Wells, 210 to Hanger, and 30 to Spooner and Harris; ARMS records show no evidence that Strasser and Callahan received any orders. ARMS records suggest that about 430 legs were actually furnished to soldiers, approximately 330 from Wells and 100 from Hanger. Although navy men were eligible for limbs, all approved orders were for applicants who had been in the army, with almost 90 percent being enlisted men. Most of the officers applying for limbs were lieutenants or captains, but applicants included one surgeon, John Henry Britts, wounded by artillery while on duty in a Vicksburg hospital, and Brigadier General Henry Harrison Walker, wounded at Spotsylvania. About 10 percent of applicants were men whose amputation had been performed by Union surgeons.[34]

Many factors contributed to ARMS being unable to supply more than a small fraction of the desired limbs. It got started late in the war, had to rely on private funding, and was not initially considered important enough to merit the assignment of large numbers of detailed conscripts or other types of government assistance. The South had no preexisting artificial-limb industry to speak of, and the experience of those that contracted with ARMS paled in comparison with the larger and much more seasoned Northern companies. Materials for making limbs got progressively scarcer and more expensive. At one point, in fall 1864, both Wells and Hanger were "compelled to suspend all operations on account of military operations in their immediate vicinity."[35]

Numerous other factors explained what success ARMS did have. Carrington worked selflessly and, with the blessing Surgeon General Moore, wielded the considerable influence he held as the officer in charge of Virginia hospitals. Wells, Hanger, and shoemaker Taylor labored faithfully while making little or no profit. Citizens, from the wealthy to those with only modest means, contributed generously.

For a private organization with peaceful aims, ARMS came to involve a surprisingly prominent—and sometimes notorious—array of personalities, including politicians, illustrious generals, a British lord, and even a deceased Union cavalryman. In the end, though, the good intentions and sacrifices that sustained ARMS could not overcome a wartime environment that was anything but conducive to the association's success.

7

Magnificent Benefaction

It is proper that the mutilated men who have received Limbs
on *Government* order, and the *public*, so largely interested in
the subject, should now learn the true and complete history of
the Nation's magnificent benefaction, tendered to its gallant
defenders.

—B. Frank. Palmer, *Report of the Great
National Benefaction*, 1868

A telling news item appeared on the front page of Atlanta's *Southern
Confederacy* on December 28, 1862. An artificial leg had been invented by Alexander George of that city. The device—the inventor's "first
effort"—displayed "remarkable mechanical genius" and had been fit to a
soldier whose leg had been amputated. "The great demand for artificial
limbs," concluded the story, "will doubtless call forth a degree of mechanical skill which may prove alike surprising and valuable."[1]

By that date, the U.S. government had already begun issuing artificial
legs to military amputees, and the South was still thirteen months away
from establishing its own program. Before George's initial foray into limb
making was being touted in Atlanta, no fewer that fourteen Northern
limb manufacturers, many with patents and long-established businesses,
had expressed a desire to furnish their devices to the Union program.

In addition to a late start and the absence of well-established limb
manufacturers, other factors—many related to the Confederacy's dete-
riorating military and economic situation—distinguished the Southern
limb program from its Northern counterpart. The lack of action by the
Confederate Congress prompted civilians to form ARMS, which relied
primarily on private donations rather than on government appropriations
like those that funded the Union program. ARMS's financial straits even
forced its officers to engage in cotton trading and put up their own money

to cover budget shortfalls. As military duty claimed able-bodied men, major contractors Wells and Hanger found themselves chronically short of skilled labor. Inflation forced prices ever higher for the raw materials they needed, such as wood, hides, and steel. Curtailment of trade with the North and an increasingly effective Union naval blockade meant that even basic necessities for crafting limbs, such as eyelets, glue, screws, files, and hacksaw blades, could not be had locally at reasonable prices.

Knowledge about artificial limbs was scarce in the South. ARMS administrator Carrington knew little about the devices, and if his fellow ARMS officers had any expertise in the subject, they seemed not to share it with him. Thus, Carrington educated himself and tirelessly sought out potential limb makers and information about limb design. When he learned that a Northern-made artificial limb had been removed from a slain Union cavalryman, he eagerly sought possession of it.

Carrington, whether he believed it or not, asserted that craftsmen such as watchmakers and gunsmiths could easily fashion satisfactory artificial limbs if given detailed drawings. He implored men with little or no limb-making experience to consult Northern patent drawings and try their hand at the task, and he seriously entertained proposals from prospective makers whose qualifications were dubious at best. Among the Southern limb makers was a man who had, only four years before, referred to himself as a wheelwright and another who had recently built gun carriages and molded grapeshot and canister balls. Carrington seemed not to believe—or could not bring himself to acknowledge—that skills other than expert craftsmanship were needed to ensure that an artificial limb had the proper fit and design to suit a patient's particular needs.[2]

U.S. surgeon general Hammond, on the other hand, had the luxury of consulting civilian and military surgeons, many of whom had considerable knowledge about artificial limbs. There were enough makers competing for government patronage that the program administrators could afford to be discerning. Having numerous models to evaluate side by side simplified somewhat the task of Union limb-selection panels, because the demonstrations and examinations allowed the comparative superiority of certain models to become obvious. At least two of the major Northern manufacturers were physicians and could call on their knowledge of anatomy and physiology. Others, like Palmer, could rely on the know-how gained from years of designing, crafting, fitting, repairing, and modifying limbs. Involvement in other endeavors was unusual among the major Northern limb makers. Dieterick W. Kolbe also made surgical instruments but specialized in orthopedic instruments and appliances.[3]

In spite of Carrington's hopes for Confederate limbs and his public stance that they rivaled or surpassed Northern devices in quality, the wartime limbs of Wells, and especially of Hanger, almost certainly failed to measure up to their Northern counterparts. Not only would this have been entirely expected—even the seasoned Northern makers would have been hampered by conditions in the Confederacy—it was borne out by Carrington's own complaints about poor materials and workmanship in Wells and Hanger limbs. The dispatching of Surgeon Darby to Europe—only fourteen months before the formation of ARMS—to secure limbs for important Confederate officers was a tacit acknowledgment that high-quality devices could not be obtained in the South. Moreover, when an 1866 panel of Southern physicians, many of whom had been Confederate surgeons (including former limbs inspector James Cabell), evaluated models of legs from twenty-three makers "for the guidance of all Physicians," the Northern devices were judged best; the legs of Wells and Hanger, although entered for consideration, were not among the nine proclaimed to be "of superior merit."[4]

Recipients of ARMS-supplied limbs were never expected to pay an additional fee, and the Southern limb manufacturers worked more directly with Carrington than the Northern makers did with the U.S. surgeon general. Carrington, although frustrated at times with Wells and Hanger, never seemed to question their basic honesty or commitment to assisting wounded soldiers. In the U.S. program, Surgeons General Hammond and Barnes and especially Surgeon Tripler became indignant with what they regarded as extortionate behavior by some limb makers. Accusations of improper charges assessed against patients may have arisen, in part, because a layer of confusion was added when recipients were given the option of paying out of pocket for higher grade models than those specified by the government. Moreover, the employment of agents by some Union suppliers, like Palmer, provided an opportunity for unscrupulous middlemen to add charges.

For all their differences, the Union and Confederate programs had much in common. Both were fortunate to have energetic army surgeons as chief administrators, and those individuals, not content to simply accept the products of the lowest bidder, paid considerable attention to quality. Both programs appreciated the importance of minimizing the distance that beneficiaries had to travel to be fitted for limbs. ARMS dealt with this by seeking manufacturers based in different regions of the Confederacy, whereas Surgeon General Hammond initially forced the approved Union suppliers, all headquartered in the East, to find ways to process orders originating at various points throughout the Union. Both programs further eased the burden on limb applicants by providing them with free transportation and lodging when they were being fitted.

In both North and South, there were similar disagreements about the type of artificial legs that should be provided. The great New York surgeon Samuel Gross, a member of the first Union panel convened to recommend prostheses, believed that peg legs would be most suitable because of their durability and economy. The board members of ARMS thought the same, although their views were probably influenced by the scarcity of experienced Southern limb makers. The manufacturers Palmer (in the North) and Wells (in the South), at least, were vocal about the inadequacy of peg legs, and both programs quickly excluded those crude devices from further consideration.

In light of all the disadvantages faced by ARMS, its actual output, in numbers of limbs provided, was well beyond what might have been expected. In the fifteen or so months of ARMS's existence, Wells and Hanger combined to provide about 430 legs. In contrast, from September 1862—when the U.S. program's first leg was probably provided—through December 1863, the five approved U.S. makers together furnished about 590 legs, with the giant of Northern makers, Palmer, supplying about 180 (appendix B). During comparable lengths of time as the respective programs got started, Southerner Wells was about twice as productive as Palmer, and Southerner Hanger was at least as productive as Northerners Hudson, Bly, and Selpho.

To be sure, Wells and Hanger were operating at full capacity and devoting their full attention to ARMS orders, whereas the Northern companies' output during the first year of the Union program was well below their limit, as proven by their increased production later in the war. Furthermore, the Northern companies continued providing limbs to the public. Nevertheless, the fact that ARMS rivaled the Union program in initial output is remarkable and a testament to the tireless work of Carrington in getting applications processed and his contractors Wells and Hanger in making the limbs. Rapidly worsening conditions in the South would have prevented the ARMS contractors from improving or even maintaining their initial performance, but one must wonder how much better ARMS could have done had it been established earlier in the war.

The end of the war opened a vast new market for Northern manufacturers, many of whom began advertising in Southern publications or establishing offices in the former Confederate states. The 1866 issues of the *Richmond Medical Journal* and the *Southern Journal of Medical*

Sciences, for example, included advertisements from Union suppliers Bly, Clement, Gildea, Hudson, Kimball, Kolbe, Marks, Palmer, Selpho, and Edward Spellerberg; from two firms, Douglass and Weston, whose devices had been deemed unsuitable for the Union program; and from Baltimore makers Henery D. Reinhardt and George Leacock, the latter yet another former employee of Palmer.

Many advertisements contained endorsements by Union army surgeons and testimonials from former Union soldiers, but some limb companies kept possible Southern sensitivities in mind. Henry Gildea of Philadelphia, for example, listed former Confederate surgeons Josiah C. Nott and Hunter Holmes McGuire as references. A single Palmer advertisement featured testimonials from five Southerners, four of whom had been Confederate army officers. In an 1868 promotional pamphlet, Richard Clement of Philadelphia listed as a reference a South Carolina physician who had formerly taught at Charleston College. Clement's pamphlet also featured as his first testimonial a letter from former Confederate general Richard S. Ewell, who had praised the Wells leg that he had worn during the war. Other prominent testimonials in Clement's pamphlet were from two former members of the 13th Virginia Cavalry.[5]

Palmer had opened an office in New Orleans during the war and continued his presence there after the war by arranging with New Orleans druggist James Syme to be his sole agent for Louisiana, Mississippi, and Texas. By late 1865, Benjamin W. Jewett had moved his headquarters from New Hampshire to Washington, D.C., and set up additional offices in Macon, Richmond, New Orleans, and Raleigh. By the next year, E. D. Hudson had opened an office in Richmond under the charge of apothecary Powhatan E. Dupuy, and Douglas Bly had established offices in New Orleans, Memphis, and Augusta, Georgia.[6]

Besides Wells and Hanger, other Southern companies, some of them new, also vied for a share of business in the former Confederate states. William T. Cole, who had unsuccessfully applied for an ARMS contract, advertised in July 1865 that he was manufacturing artificial arms and legs at Newman, Georgia. By mid-1866, Dannelly, Marshall and Company, with former Confederate surgeon Francis Olin Dannelly as senior partner, was operating branches of New York's National Leg and Arm Company in Madison, Georgia; Columbia, South Carolina; and Nashville. The firm, which used designs patented by Thomas Uren of New York, employed "disabled soldiers in their various factories—paying a fair amount to beginners," but nevertheless assured potential Madison customers that "our workmen are the most skilled, from the Company in New York." The

Madison branch was called the Southern Leg and Arm Company. Another former Confederate surgeon, Harvey Leonides Byrd, obtained a U.S. patent for an artificial leg and opened a business in Augusta, Georgia.[7]

Confederate veterans were ineligible to receive artificial limbs or other benefits from the U.S. government, so within a few years after the war's end, a number of Southern states established programs to assist their amputees. In 1866, for example, North Carolina provided New Hampshire limb maker Benjamin W. Jewett with a building in Raleigh for the manufacture of artificial legs, for which the state paid $70 each. Disabled former soldiers traveling to Raleigh for a prosthesis were provided with free transportation and lodging; those who had already purchased a limb could receive cash commutation. Jewett's productivity was initially hampered by an inefficient workforce and problems obtaining materials, but he managed to turn out 221 legs—the state estimated that about 550 were needed—in the first seven months of the program. The superintendent of the state's artificial limb department declared that most of Jewett's limbs had "proven entirely satisfactory." The problems that did arise were "owing to the very peculiar formation of the stumps of the parties, and to their unwillingness or inability to . . . return to this place if their limbs are inefficient, either because of a bad fit, or the weakness of the machinery." In June of the next year, Jewett's workshop closed for lack of work.[8]

The legs made by Douglas Bly were selected for the artificial limbs programs of Virginia, South Carolina, and Georgia; Virginia also designated James E. Hanger as a supplier. South Carolina paid Bly $74.65 for his model without lateral ankle motion and allowed for beneficiaries to pay an extra $75.35 out of pocket if they desired the lateral-motion model. South Carolina's governor, James L. Orr, declared that Bly had "faithfully complied with his contract, and that the legs furnished by him have been substantial and given very general satisfaction." In compliance with an act of March 12, 1866, Georgia contracted in September 1866 with Bly to supply in Macon his legs without lateral ankle motion for $70 each. He was also to furnish arms—of the patent by New York City's Jonathan H. Koeller—for $70 or $40, depending on whether the amputation was above or below the elbow, and to stop when the total cost for all limbs reached $20,000. Disabled soldiers who were excluded by exhaustion of the 1866 appropriation could apply, starting in early 1867, for the Eureka Artificial Leg, invented by Georgian Harvey L. Byrd and made in partnership with Dieterick H. Kolbe of Philadelphia—or for Kolbe's artificial arm, made by Kolbe alone.[9]

Alabama, Arkansas, Florida, and Mississippi also enacted legislation in 1866 or 1867 to provide Southern amputees with artificial limbs. In the absence of similar government action in Louisiana during the immediate postwar period, a ladies' benevolent society in that state raised money to buy limbs and provide other assistance to the state's soldiers and their survivors. Similar organizations arose elsewhere. The Benevolent Society of Tennessee, for example, and the Ladies' Tennessee Benevolent Association helped pay for limbs in that state. In later years, former Confederate states enacted or extended legislation that provided military amputees with artificial limbs or cash commutation.[10]

For former U.S. military personnel, legislation in 1870 allowed veterans who had previously received an artificial limb or apparatus for resection to receive a new device or the money value instead—$75 for an artificial leg or $50 for an arm, foot, or resection apparatus—as soon as practicable and then every five years thereafter. In 1872, benefits were extended to include not only amputees but individuals who had "sustained bodily injuries [not necessarily amputations] depriving them of the use of any of their limbs," and free transportation for the purpose of fitting devices was granted. In 1891, Congress reduced the allowed frequency of device replacement or commutation from every five to every three years. The Senate Committee on Military Affairs supported this change after determining that although the average artificial limb might last five years, its average annual repair cost was $25—this in spite of the fact that manufacturers were obliged "to make good for five years all defects of materials or workmanship without additional charge." According to manufacturer A. A. Marks, the change "was not done because soldiers required new limbs so frequently, but as an additional gratuity to the maimed."[11]

Starting in 1870, applications for U.S. benefits increased steadily as veterans whose arms or legs were injured during the war, but not amputated, found that age and the effects of disease made those limbs progressively less usable. Thus, reported the surgeon general in 1892, veterans "who had comparatively good use of their limbs in 1870 are now completely disabled." Applications increased markedly in two waves before 1891. The first reflected the activity of pension claim agents, who for a 10-percent commission, assisted veterans in obtaining commutation payments. The second resulted from the surgeon general's efforts to inform potential beneficiaries that applying was simple enough not to require agents.[12]

Disabled Union veterans overwhelmingly chose to receive money in place of a new limb or resection device. For the year ending in June 1871, the first twelve months during which amputees could apply for reissue of a limb or commutation, 104 beneficiaries opted for a new arm, whereas 4,067 took the payment instead. Artificial legs were selected by 1,117 veterans, while 3,114 chose commutation. Out of 560 applicants eligible for a resection apparatus, 538 settled for the payment. By 1892, about 10,000 amputees had been approved for benefits and, on average, each had applied successfully about four times for a new limb or commutation since 1870. During those years, arm amputees chose a new device over commutation only 1.4 percent of the time, and leg amputees selected a new leg 21.9 percent of the time.[13]

The same phenomenon occurred in the South. In 1872 and 1873 combined, for example, Virginia paid James E. Hanger for furnishing 142 artificial limbs but issued 432 commutation payments. In 1888 and 1889 combined, Louisiana paid for 20 artificial legs and issued 124 commutation payments for the loss of an arm or leg.[14]

The usefulness of an artificial arm, said the U.S. surgeon general in 1892, "is regarded as nil, and although some may claim it to be an ornamental addition to a maimed individual, the man with a war record generally prefers his empty sleeve." Even those veterans who had been issued an artificial arm almost always opted for commutation the next time they applied for benefits. Legislation allowed amputees free round-trip transportation—including, according to the secretary of war, "sleeping car accommodations on occasion of night travel"—to visit the manufacturer of their choice for fitting, "thus affording an opportunity," remarked the surgeon general, "to those who had settled in the West to have a trip to New York, Philadelphia, or other eastern city which might be utilized in seeing old friend and relatives." Even this inducement, though, was not enough for most amputees to forgo the commutation payment. "The artificial leg," the surgeon general continued, "is shown by the statistics to be an appliance of much more practical value than the arm," and the high rate of commutation for leg amputations, he thought, reflected in part the large number of beneficiaries who had to select payment because their stump did not allow the wearing of an artificial leg. Moreover, "the financial circumstances of many of the old soldiers are such as to prevent them from accepting the expensive luxury of an artificial leg when its acceptance would cause them the loss of the $75 which they would otherwise obtain." The very high overall rate of commutation payments could also have been explained by the issued limbs not needing repair or replacement, but given that only 4,421 artificial legs were issued to 5,134 U.S. veterans from 1870 to 1892, the devices would had to have been very durable indeed.[15]

The fact that amputees so frequently favored commutation payments over new artificial limbs casts doubt on the wisdom of the wartime programs. Perhaps those efforts should instead have provided amputees with peg legs or only monetary payments; doing so would certainly have saved much time. There was, however, a widespread belief that the best available articulated artificial limbs were triumphs of human ingenuity and craftsmanship, and the limb makers themselves helped convince program administrators that this notion was correct. In light of the huge sacrifice that military amputees had made for their country, politicians and the public—and even the amputees themselves—might have thought it improper to provide anything but what was thought to be the best. The many wartime applications for limbs suggest that amputees at first thought the limbs worth trying, especially since commutation was not allowed at the time, and their opinions of the devices' value may have changed once they used them, observed the experiences of other amputees, or found themselves in financial difficulties.

In spite of veterans' tendency to turn down artificial limbs, activity in the limbs industry itself continued to grow. Not only did the number of patents increase after the war, so did the number of companies, a trend attributable more to the large number of railroad and other accidents than to demand by Civil War veterans; a single 1893 issue of a monthly magazine for railroad workers had advertisements from eighteen limb companies. According to one historian, the United States had 200 limb manufacturers in 1917. Of the Northern makers active during the Civil War, one of the most successful and long-lasting was the A. A. Marks Company, which by 1888 was calling itself the largest manufacturer in the country. Marks was bought in 1957 by the Winkley Artificial Limb Company, which was founded in 1888 and exists today as Winkley Orthotics and Prosthetics. Meanwhile, the business started by Virginian James E. Hanger expanded, thrived, and continues today as Hanger Orthopedic Group, which provides orthotic and prosthetic devices and operates several hundred care centers in the United States.[16]

As Civil War limb companies can be linked to the present, so too can the Union and Confederate artificial-limbs programs. The U.S. program was the first government endeavor to offer artificial limbs to wounded soldiers and sailors, and ARMS was the only Confederacy-wide attempt to provide similar assistance to wounded Southerners. During the war, the sheer numbers of sick and wounded military men limited the assistance that either North or South could provide. Amputees receiving a limb from either program could get assistance from the issuing organization if they had problems with the device's fit or quality. In the North, the U.S. Sanitary Commission supplemented the government's wartime activities by providing information about the limbs programs, lodging amputees who were traveling to obtain a limb, operating convalescent homes for discharged soldiers, and advocating for more generous pensions—and the return of disabled service members to their communities—as an alternative to military asylums and soldiers' homes. Rehabilitative services as they exist today—physical, occupational, and recreational therapy, for example—were absent. Other than pension payments and periodic offerings of a replacement limb or a commutation payment, a veteran with an artificial limb could not look to the government for assistance in mastering his prosthesis, finding a job, or dealing with the other difficulties that attended his injury.[17]

Since that time, care for military amputees has become a more all-encompassing and cooperative effort involving multiple organizations, some of them civilian-based, and emphasizing a holistic approach to medical treatment and rehabilitation. This evolution has been influenced by multiple factors, including the types of wounds suffered in various conflicts, increased understanding of and ability to address the multifaceted needs of patients, and advances in treatment and technology. Limb amputation has become an all-too-common outcome of wounds sustained in the current global war on terror, occurring in more than 900 American service members by mid-2009. The special needs of those amputees, including for many a desire to return to active duty, has led to the development of a comprehensive, sophisticated, and multidisciplinary amputee care program that requires close teamwork between the Department of Defense and the Department of Veterans Affairs and the assistance of public and private organizations.[18]

There were pragmatic motives behind the Civil War's artificial limbs programs. Much better, said advocates of the Union effort, to provide amputees with artificial limbs and enable them to earn a living than to let them become a burden on society. The promise of limbs for the maimed might also have made enlisting in the military more palatable. Yet when William Carrington described the plight of maimed soldiers and sailors "hobbling on wooden pegs, or swinging on the galling crutch," he got to the crux of the issue: Young men were sustaining grievous wounds for their country, and they deserved whatever assistance could be provided to help them return to a more normal life. The program administrators, many of them long-term military men as well as physicians, must have understood instinctively their duty to aid their countrymen and fellow service members, and the same feeling of obligation no doubt moved other key participants—from legislators and contractors to private donors—to assist in their own way. As expressions of esteem, gratitude, and humanity, the Union and Confederate programs quickly provided beneficiaries with some of the best devices that could be obtained.[19]

Although much has changed since the Civil War, the hard work, sacrifice, and benevolent motives of those seeking to assist amputees have not. The wartime Union and Confederate efforts, when considered with the postwar federal and state programs, represent first steps in the government's and society's ongoing commitment to the care and rehabilitation of its military amputees. The dedicated individuals who played a part in the artificial-limbs programs some 150 years ago would regard with pride their contribution to today's state-of-the-art amputee care program for American service members.

APPENDIXES

NOTES

BIBLIOGRAPHY

INDEX

Appendix A.
Makers and Inventors Associated with the Union and Confederate Artificial-Limbs Programs

The artificial-limb makers and inventors listed here were candidates to supply the U.S. limbs program through 1865, the Confederacy's Association for the Relief of Maimed Soldiers (ARMS), or the individual state programs in the South through 1867. The surgeon general of the U.S. Army convened four major boards of surgeons during the war to evaluate large numbers of candidate limbs: in August–September 1862, October 1863, July–August 1864, and March 1865 (hereafter called the 1862, 1863, 1864, and 1865 U.S. boards). Other U.S. boards met from time to time to evaluate one or a few models. A board of Southern physicians met in Richmond, Virginia, in 1866 (hereafter called the 1866 Richmond board) to evaluate a large number of artificial arms and legs. Since its presumed aim was, at least in part, to provide recommendations that could be adopted by individual Southern states as they established their own postwar programs, the makers evaluated by that board are also included below.

Additional information about many of the makers can be found elsewhere in this book, with documentation provided in the associated notes. For this appendix, documentation is provided for only the information that does not appear elsewhere. Makers and inventors that do not appear elsewhere are indicated by an asterisk (*).

American Arm and Leg Company. Based in Washington, D.C., the American Arm and Leg Company's president was Willard Bliss, M.D., a former U.S. Army surgeon who had attended at the bedside of both Presidents Lincoln and Garfield after they were mortally wounded. A board of surgeons evaluated the company's artificial leg in December 1865 and concluded that "the limb as a whole presents no special advantages over those already authorized for issue." The leg was nevertheless approved in late January 1866 for the U.S. program, and the 1866 board judged the company's leg eighth best among those presented by twenty-three companies. The company's leg appears to have been of the pattern patented by James Walber in 1865.[1]

American Artificial Limb Company. * *See* Palmer, Benjamin Franklin

American Leg Company. *See* Small and McMillen

Bly, Douglas, M.D. Bly, headquartered in Rochester, New York, was one of the first makers selected to furnish limbs for the Union artificial-limbs program. He was especially known for his leg with lateral ankle movement. His limbs were also selected by at least three postwar programs in the former Confederate states. U.S.

patents 17,888 (leg, with R. H. Nicholas, 1857), 23,656 (leg, 1859), 24,062 (leg, 1859), 25,238 (leg, 1859), 31,438 (leg, 1861), 38,549 (leg, 1863), 38,550 (leg, 1863), 57,666 (leg, 1866), and 87,264 (leg, 1869).

Bradley, William. Bradley, an agent for the Manchester Cotton Mills in Virginia, made an artificial leg for General Richard Ewell and submitted an artificial arm to William Carrington of ARMS. Carrington approved of the arm and ordered one but did not make a contract with Bradley.

Brenner, Peter.* Brenner, of Augusta, Georgia, was identified by William Carrington of ARMS as a person who had made artificial limbs but was "not extensively engaged in their manufacture." Although Carrington presumably explored the possibility of doing business with Brenner, ARMS records do not so indicate.[2]

Brown, William F.* Brown, of Amherst County, Virginia, was identified by William Carrington of ARMS as a person who had made artificial limbs but was "not extensively engaged in their manufacture." Although Carrington presumably explored the possibility of doing business with Browns, ARMS records do not so indicate.[3]

Byrd, Harvey Leonides. Byrd, a former Confederate surgeon, patented a leg in 1866, opened an office in Augusta, Georgia, and presented his device to the 1866 Richmond board, which did not deem it among the top nine entries. Byrd's Eureka leg, made in collaboration with Dieterick W. Kolbe, was approved for Georgia veterans starting in 1867. An 1868 U.S. board was unimpressed with Byrd's leg and did not recommend it. U.S. patent 52,964 (leg, 1866).[4]

Clement, Richard. Clement knew B. Frank. Palmer in New Hampshire before Palmer fashioned his first artificial leg in 1846 and was one of Palmer's first workmen. Clement claimed to have made the Palmer models that won acclaim at the Great Exhibition in London. Clement started his own business in Philadelphia by 1860 and was approved as a supplier for the Union limb program in May 1865 after a favorable showing before the 1865 U.S. board. U.S. patent 47,281 (leg, 1865).

Cole, William T. Cole, of Columbus, Georgia, expressed interest in supplying artificial legs for ARMS, but his devices, while considered to have "suitable properties," were more expensive than the organization was willing to pay. He did not receive a contract. Advertisements from Cole appeared in Georgia newspapers in 1866.

Condell, John. Condell, of Morristown, New York, submitted an artificial arm and leg for consideration by the 1865 U.S. board. The arm was approved in May 1865, but no Condell arms were furnished by May 1866. U.S. patents 48,659 (arm, 1865), 48,660 (leg, 1865), and 48,792 (leg, 1865).

Cotty, Edward. Cotty, of Washington, D.C., presented an artificial arm to the 1863 U.S. board. The device was "clumsy in appearance," and the hand, made of pure German silver, was heavy. Cotty said that he would be replacing the metal hand with one made of vulcanized rubber. The model was not recommended for approval. U.S. patent 40,397 (arm, 1863).[5]

Daniels, Phylander. An artificial leg made of leather was presented by Daniels of New York City for evaluation by the 1864 U.S. board. It was not approved then or at any time during the war. U.S. patents 37,738 (artificial-leg support, 1863) and 41,282 (leg, 1864).

Davis, Levi G. Davis, of Fluvanna County, Virginia, formed a business with William B. Hodgson manufacturing artificial limbs. He was invited in March 1864 by William Carrington of ARMS to submit a model but suggested that he had more business than he could manage. He is not known to have furnished limbs for ARMS.

Douglass, Darwin DeForrest. Douglass was a workman for B. Frank. Palmer before opening his own business in Springfield, Massachusetts. He was erroneously reported in 1862 to be one of the makers chosen to supply artificial legs to the Union program but was never so selected during the war. U.S. patent 26,753 (leg, 1860).

Drake, John S. An early leg design patented by Drake, while he was in New York City, was unusual in being partially composed of whalebone. Headquartered in Boston, Drake entered a leg for consideration by the 1862 U.S. board, but it was not approved. At the time, Drake's agent in New York was George Tiemann and Company, a major supplier of surgical instruments. The 1865 Union board also declined to recommend Drake's arms and leg. U.S. patents 9,232 (leg, 1852), 15,372 (hand and arm, 1856), and 57,691 (leg, 1866).[6]

Engelbrecht, Theodore F. Engelbrecht, of New York City, patented an artificial leg of "corrugated plate metal" with Reinhold Boeklen and William Staehlen of Brooklyn. Engelbrecht presented a model of corrugated brass to the 1862 Union board, but it was not recommended. In 1863, legs of Engelbrecht's design were being sold by J. W. Weston. U.S. patent 37,282 (leg, 1863).[7] *See* Weston, James W.

Foster, James A. Foster, an amputee, worked for an artificial-limb maker before designing the Patent Union Artificial Limb and opening an office in Detroit. His artificial leg was considered but not recommended by the 1865 U.S. board. By 1868, Foster had additional offices in Philadelphia, Cincinnati, and Rochester, New York, and was making artificial arms of the patent owned by the National Leg and Arm Company. U.S. patents 49,253 (leg, 1865) and 92,031 (leg, 1869).[8]

Fravel, John. After learning of the recommendations of the 1862 U.S. board, Fravel of St. Louis asked for an opportunity to have his artificial leg considered. He was invited to submit a model, but if he did, it was not recommended for approval during the war. U.S. patent 39,912 (leg, 1863).

Gildea, Henry A. Gildea, headquartered in Philadelphia, made both artificial arms and legs. His legs were not approved for the wartime Union limbs program, but in May 1863, his arms became only the second approved, after Selpho's. He appears not to have patented any of his designs.

Grenell, Increase M. An artificial arm and leg were presented to the 1864 U.S. board by I. M. Grenell and Company of New York City. The board found the brass leg (George L. Shepard's patent) undesirable and declined to recommend it. Grenell offered to supply the limbs "made either of metal gutta percha or hide." The arm (Jonathan H. Koeller's patents) was considered insufficiently tested at that time but was approved in January 1865. U.S. patent 42,799 (Shepard, leg, 1864). *See* Koeller, Jonathan H.[9]

Hall, George W.[*] Hall, of Buffalo, submitted a model leg to the 1865 U.S. board, but it was not recommended by that panel. U.S. patent 38,739 (leg, 1863).[10]

Hanger, James Edward. Hanger, from Staunton, Virginia, was one of two major suppliers for ARMS. He was one of the first amputees of the Civil War and formed Hanger and Brother with his brother John M. Hanger. James had the first two Confederate patents for artificial limbs. His company exists today as the Hanger Orthopedic Group. Confederate patents 155 (leg, 1863) and 201 (leg, 1863). U.S. patent 111,741 (leg, 1871).

Hudson, Erasmus Darwin, M.D. Hudson bought an interest in B. Frank. Palmer's artificial-leg patent in the late 1840s and, by 1860, helped manage Palmer's branches in New York City and New England. He established his own company in New York City, which was one of the first selected to supply artificial legs for the Union program. He was accused by Palmer of patent violation. Hudson had a particular interest in apparatus for limb resection. He did not patent any of his devices.

Hughes and Knode.[*] The firm of Hughes and Knode, of Montgomery, Alabama, was identified by William Carrington of ARMS as a "regular" manufacturer of artificial limbs. Carrington presumably explored the possibility of contracting with the firm, but ARMS records do not so indicate.[11]

Jewett, Benjamin W. Jewett worked for B. Frank. Palmer in New Hampshire, having known Palmer since the late 1840s. He established his own firm in New Hampshire before moving to Washington, D.C., after he was selected in 1862 to furnish legs for the Union program. Jewett was repeatedly accused by Palmer of patent violation. He was selected to provide limbs for the North Carolina program after the war. U.S. patents 16,360 (leg, 1857) and 29,494 (leg, 1860).

Jewett, George Baker. A minister and amputee, G. B. Jewett invented an artificial leg of novel design and established a company in Salem, Massachusetts. The device was called the Salem leg to distinguish it from the limbs of Benjamin W. Jewett, who was evidently unrelated. The Salem leg was approved for the Union program in May 1865. U.S. patents 35,686 (leg, 1862), 35,937 (leg, 1862), 44,534 (leg, 1864), 49,528 (leg, 1865), 49,529 (leg, 1865), and 51,593 (leg, 1865).[12]

Kimball and Lawrence. Hiram A. Kimball and Andrew J. Lawrence of Philadelphia submitted models of artificial arms and legs to the 1864 Union board. The leg, made of hard rubber, was considered not sufficiently tested and thus not recommended. The board considered the arm good but not sturdy enough and declined to recommend it. A leg and arm from Kimball (Lawrence was not mentioned) were approved in May 1866. U.S. patents 39,578 (Kimball, hand, 1863), 47,835 (Kimball and Lawrence, arm, 1865), and 54,364 (Kimball and Lawrence, leg, 1866).

Koeller, Jonathan H. Inventor Koeller, of New York City, evidently did not apply directly to become a supplier to the U.S. program or to a postwar Southern program, but arms of his design, as made by I. M. Grenell, were approved for the U.S. program in January 1865. Koeller-designed arms, as made by Douglas Bly, were approved in 1866 for the Georgia program. U.S. patents 43,590 (arm, 1864) and 44, 638 (arm, 1864).

Kolbe, Dieterick W. Kolbe, of Philadelphia, presented models of arms and legs to the 1862 Union board, but they were not approved. His arms were approved in August 1864. Kolbe was also a manufacturer of medical instruments. U.S. patent 45,052 (arm, 1864).

Leacock, George. In 1866, Leacock, of Baltimore, boasted of fourteen years of experience working with B. Frank. Palmer and presented his artificial leg to the 1866 Richmond board, which did not recognize it as one of the nine best.[13]

Lincoln, Marvin. Lincoln held a one-third interest in the New England and New York City branches of B. Frank. Palmer's company in the late 1850s and, after selling his interest, was foreman of Palmer's Boston branch. Lincoln opened his own establishment in New York City for the manufacture and sale of artificial arms and was one of the early makers approved to supply arms for the Union limbs program. Lincoln and Palmer furnished artificial limbs through the same office during the war. U.S. patent 39,478 (arm, 1863).[14]

Lockie, Peter. Lockie, of Rochester, New York, submitted an artificial arm and leg for consideration by the 1865 Union board. The board did not recommend them. U.S. patent 40,417 (leg, 1863).[15]

Marks, Amasa Abraham. A. A. Marks began making artificial limbs in 1853 and became best known for making solid rubber feet and hands. Based in New York, the Marks Company did not become an approved Union supplier until May 1865. In the decades following the war, A. A. Marks claimed to be the largest artificial-limb company in the country. Promotional efforts included numerous editions of books written by George E. Marks, who along with A. A. Marks and William A. Marks, constituted the firm of A. A. Marks. U.S. patents 40,763 (1863, leg) and 46,687 (1865, leg).[16]

Matlack, Mason W. During the Civil War, Matlack, an amputee from Philadelphia, made and sold the metallic skeleton leg patented by George W. Yerger although not an approved Union supplier during the war. Matlack's leg was presented to but not recommended by the 1865 U.S. board.

Mayo, Littleton Upshur. Mayo, of Pattonsburg or Buchanon, Virginia, served as a Confederate surgeon but was dismissed after a court-martial. He offered to manufacture large numbers of artificial legs, purportedly an improvement on Palmer's model, for ARMS. He did not become a contractor for ARMS.

Miller, J. A., Dr. J. (or I.) Miller of New York City presented an artificial leg to the 1864 U.S. board, which declined to consider it because of uncertainty about its ownership and a disagreement between Miller and a firm called Miller and Wells, also of New York City. *See* Miller, W. H.

Miller, W. H.* Written material from Dr. W. H. Miller of New York City was presented to the 1863 U.S. board, but that board's report did not mention this individual. He may have been the Dr. J. or I. Miller mentioned in the report.[17]

Miller and Wells. Individuals named Miller and Wells separately presented artificial arms to the 1863 U.S. board. The models were almost identical and were not recommended by the board. A firm called Miller and Wells, of New York City, presented an artificial leg to the 1864 U.S. board, which declined to consider it because of uncertainty about its ownership and a disagreement between the firm and Dr. J. (or I.) Miller. Wells may have been Charles Wells.[18]

Monroe and Gardiner. Joshua Monroe and Jetur Gardiner operated a firm in New York City for the production of artificial legs made of "imperishable rawhide." The devices were considered but not recommended for the Union limbs program in 1864 and 1865. They were finally approved for the program in May 1866. U.S. patents 41,934 (leg, 1864), 44,644 (leg, 1864), and 49,038 (leg, 1865).[19]

National Leg and Arm Company. Manufacturers Chauncey A. Frees and Thomas Gilmore of New York produced artificial limbs of Thomas Uren's design for the National Leg and Arm Company, whose president was William Henry Tiffany. The 1865 Union board did not recommend approval of the firm's leg or apparatus for resection, but upon the board's advice, the arm was approved in May 1865. A panel reexamining the leg in June 1866 thought it was no better than already approved legs and had "a somewhat inferior mechanical finish." Shortly after the war, the company opened branches of the same name in Columbia, South Carolina, and in Nashville, with another branch in Madison, Georgia, called the Southern Leg and Arm Company.[20]

Ord, John F. *See* Yerger, George W.

Palmer, Benjamin Franklin. The artificial limbs of B. Frank. Palmer were probably the best known of the Civil War era and were the standard against which others were judged. Palmer, an amputee, started his business in 1846 in New Hampshire. During the war, his main office was in Philadelphia, although he had branches in New York, Boston, and elsewhere. Palmer was among the five leg makers first chosen to supply the Union limbs program in 1862 and furnished legs, and later arms, throughout the rest of the war. In 1864, he became president of the newly formed American Artificial Limb Company, which purchased his former business, and by 1868, Palmer repurchased the patents and stock and ran the company personally. Numerous limb companies were formed by men who had worked with or for Palmer. U.S. patents 4,834 (1846, leg), 6,122 (1849, leg), 9,200 (1852, leg), 22,576 (1859, arm and hand), and 137,711 (1873, leg).[21]

Phillips, L. D.* Phillips, of New York City, presented an artificial arm to the 1865 U.S. board; it was not recommended. No other details about Phillips have been found.[22]

Reichenbach, John.* Reichenbach, from Pittsburgh, submitted an artificial leg for consideration by the 1865 Union board. The board did not recommend it. U.S. patents 41,237 (leg, 1864), 41,238 (leg, 1864), and 128,907 (leg, 1872).[23]

Reinhardt, Henery D. Reinhardt, of Baltimore, invented the "India rubber spring leg," advertised it in the South, and presented it to the 1866 Richmond board, which did not rank it among the top nine legs. U.S. patent 41,535 (leg, 1864).[24]

Richards and Walber.* The Newark-based firm of Richards and Walber submitted an artificial arm and leg to the 1865 Union board but did not receive the board's recommendation. Richards has not been identified. Walber may have been James Walber. *See* Walber, James[25]

Rosenstein, D. H.* Rosenstein, of St. Louis, presented an artificial arm to the 1865 U.S. board; it was not recommended. No further details about Rosenstein have been found.[26]

Rummel, Frank.* Rummel had a one-man artificial-leg shop in Augusta, Georgia. ARMS's William Carrington recognized the desirability of having a supplier in Georgia and hoped to have a maker in that part of the Confederacy produce 150 legs per month. The small size of Rummel's business and the difficulty of finding workmen prevented him from contracting with ARMS.[27]

Salem Leg Company. *See* Jewett, George Baker

Selpho, William. Selpho learned his craft in England from James Potts, inventor of the Anglesey leg, and came to the United States in 1839 to start his own business in New York City. Selpho's was the oldest firm to supply limbs, both arms and legs, for the Union program. During the war, the name of the company was changed from William Selpho to William Selpho and Son, to include his son Edwin. U.S. patents 14, 836 (leg, 1856), 18,021 (hand, 1857), and 26,378 (hand, with James Walber, 1859).

Small and McMillen. Isaac D. Small partnered with a Mr. McMillen to produce the American Artificial Leg in Cleveland. The firm, also called the American Leg Company, was approved as a Union supplier of artificial legs in December 1864 after the meeting of a special board earlier that month. It was removed from the list of suppliers after the 1865 U.S. board declined to recommend it. U.S. patent (by Small) 40,956 (leg, 1863).[28]

Southern Leg and Arm Company. The Madison, Georgia, branch of the National Leg and Arm Company was called the Southern Leg and Arm Company. It and the Columbia (South Carolina) and Nashville branches of the National Leg and Arm Company were operated by Dannelly, Marshall and Company, whose senior partner was Francis Olin Dannelly, a former Confederate surgeon. The 1866 Richmond board voted the arms made by the National Leg and Arm Company and the Southern Leg and Arm Company the best for bilateral amputation.[29]

Spellerberg, Edward. Spellerberg, of Philadelphia, did not appear on official lists of approved U.S. suppliers, but he supplied enough artificial arms in 1865 to suggest that he was indeed approved. U.S. patents 42,515 (arm, 1864) and 51,238 (arm, 1865).

Spooner and Harris. G. W. Spooner, a former employee of Wells and Brother, partnered with machinist R. F. Harris to produce artificial limbs in Charlottesville, Virginia. The design was that of Thomas R. Dolan, who had also worked for Wells. Spooner and Harris were awarded an ARMS contract, probably in January 1865. They received approximately thirty orders but appear to have delivered none.

Stafford, Charles. During the war, Stafford sold legs of Wilcox's patent though his office in Chicago. He was approved as a supplier for the Union program in 1863. *See* Wilcox, O. D.

Stoffel, Ignatius.* After the May 1865 U.S. board declined to recommend the artificial arms of Stoffel, from Washington, D.C., another board met in October 1865 to reconsider the device. Not impressed, the panelists thought the model was "roughly made" and that being made largely of metal "will be apt therefore to be soiled by secretion and corroded by the weather, while every motion is attended with an unpleasant grating sound." U.S. patents 45,876 (arm, 1865) and 57,594 (arm, 1866).[30]

Strasser, Albert. Strasser, from Montgomery, Alabama, formed a partnership with a Mr. Callahan to produce artificial legs and received a contract in December 1864 or January 1865 to provide limbs for ARMS. The firm appears not to have received any orders from ARMS. Strasser held one of three Confederate patents for artificial limbs; the other two were held by James E. Hanger. Confederate patent 252 (leg, 1864). U.S. patent 76,267 (leg, 1868).

Summersett, Christopher H. Summersett, of Wilmington, North Carolina, was dismissed as a lieutenant from a North Carolina infantry regiment for prolonged absence without leave. He submitted a model of a simple artificial leg to ARMS. He appears not to have been awarded a contract.

Tozer, Richard.* Tozer, of Columbia, South Carolina, was identified by William Carrington of ARMS as a person who had made limbs but was not extensively engaged in their manufacture. Carrington contacted Tozer but did not make a contract with him.[31]

Universal Joint and Artificial Limb Company.* *See* Weston, James W.

Uren, Thomas. Uren patented artificial upper and lower extremities when he was in San Francisco and New York City. Limbs of his design were made by the National Leg and Arm Company and its branches. U.S. patents 39,599 (leg, 1863), 46,158 (arm and hand, 1865), 46,159 (arm and hand, 1865), and 48,002 (arm, 1865).

Van Hoesen, Casper.* Van Hoesen, of New York City, submitted an artificial leg for consideration by the 1865 Union board. The board did not recommend it.[32]

Walber, James.* James Walber and Charles Wells of New York City submitted written material to the 1864 U.S. board about their artificial leg, but the board's report did not mention Walber. Walber's leg patent was evidently used by the American Arm and Leg Company. U.S. patents 26,378 (with William Selpho, hand, 1859) and 49,936 (leg, 1865).[33]

Wells, Charles.* Wells, of New York City, and James Walber of the same city submitted written material about their artificial leg to the 1864 U.S. board, but Walber was not mentioned in the board's report. A Mr. Wells was mentioned in the report of the 1863 U.S. board as presenting an arm, and a firm called Miller and Wells of New York City was mentioned in the 1864 U.S. board report as presenting a leg. *See* Miller, J. A., Dr.; Miller, W. H.; Miller and Wells; and Walber, James[34]

Wells, George W. Wells and his brother John, of Charlottesville, Virginia, formed Wells and Brother, the primary supplier of artificial limbs to ARMS. Wells furnished legs for Confederate generals Richard S. Ewell and John B. Hood.

Weston, James W. Weston offered a tinned version of a silver-plated leg to the 1864 U.S. board. It is unclear whether the design was his or perhaps that of Theodore Engelbrecht, whose model he had previously made. The board declined to recommend it. The 1865 U.S. board also declined to recommend Weston's leg. Weston called his firm the Universal Joint and Artificial Limb Company. U.S. patents 41,456 (limb socket, 1864), 45,662 (artificial-leg support, 1864), 48,138 (leg, with Thomas B. Stanley of New York, 1865), and 53,931 (leg, with Friedrick Bücher of New York and Reinhold Boeklen of Brooklyn, 1866).[35] *See* Engelbrecht, Theodore F.

Wilcox, O. D. Wilcox, of Easton, Pennsylvania, invented an artificial leg that featured a sack "of suitable material" suspended from the limb's upper edge to act as a socket. U.S. patents 15,831 (leg, 1856), and 16,420 (leg, 1857). *See* Stafford, Charles

Yerger, George W. Yerger invented the "metallic skeleton" leg and sold it with partner John F. Ord through their office in Philadelphia. During the Civil War, Philadelphia maker Mason W. Matlack sold the Yerger leg. U.S. patent 7,204 (leg, 1850).

Appendix B.
Artificial Limbs and Resection Apparatus Supplied to U.S. Soldiers and Sailors by May 10, 1866

Devices and Makers	Month Approved	Number of Devices Supplied					
		1862	1863	1864	1865	1866	Total
Legs and feet							
B. W. Jewett	Sept. 1862[1]	6	156	165	380	25	732
B. F. Palmer	Oct. 1862[2]	15	166	389	554	16	1,141[3]
E. D. Hudson	Oct.-Nov. 1862[4]	8	109	158	133	6	414
D. Bly	Nov. 1862[5]	3	79	241	518	32	873
W. Selpho	Nov. 1862,[6] Aug. 1864[7]	1	13	34	113	27	188
C. Stafford	Feb. 1863[8]	3	27	51	18	2	101
Small & McMillen	Dec. 1864[9]	...	...	0	26	0	26
R. Clement	May 1865[10]	...	1	...	74	10	85
A. A. Marks	May 1865[10]	...	...	...	44	5	49
Salem Leg Co.	May 1865[10]	...	2	5	138	11	156
Others or unspecified[11]	...	1	1	9	22	0	33
Total		37	554	1,052	2,020	134	3,798
Arms and hands							
W. Selpho	By Apr. 1863,[12] Dec. 1863[13]	...	10	67	104	2	183
H. A. Gildea	May 1863[14]	...	70	102	64	2	238
M. Lincoln	Dec. 1863[13]	...	1	349	604	52	1,006
B. F. Palmer	Dec. 1863[13]	...	1	18	37	0	56
D. W. Kolbe	Aug. 1864[7]	...	...	19	160	9	188
I. M. Grenell	Jan. 1865[15]	...	...	28	242[16]	11	281
Nat'l Leg & Arm Co.	May 1865[10]	...	...	1	81	12	94
H. A. Kimball	May 1866[17]	...	...	...	...	1	1
E. Spellerberg	Undetermined	...	...	3	141	0	144
Others or unspecified[18]	...	...	3	2	8	0	13
Total		...	85	589	1,441	89	2,204
Resection apparatus							
E. D. Hudson	By Dec. 1864[19]	...	...	6	48	3	57
D. W. Kolbe	May 1865[10]	...	...	...	20	1	21
Others[20]	...	...	...	...	11	0	11
Total		...	...	6	79	4	89
Grand total		37	639	1,647	3,540	227	6,091

Source: J. K. Barnes, Artificial Limbs Furnished to Soldiers, H.R. Exec. Doc. No. 39–108 (1st Sess. 1866).

Note: The Barnes document, which lists devices supplied by May 10, 1866, contains numerous entries indicating limbs being furnished before a maker was approved by the surgeon general or by a maker not known to have been approved. Some beneficiaries received two legs or two arms.

NOTES

The following abbreviations refer to materials at the National Archives and Records Administration (NARA), Washington, D.C.

ARMS   Record Book, Soldiers Home Hospital and the Association for the Relief of Maimed Soldiers, 1862–65 (vol. 463), Medical Department (ch. 6), War Department Collection of Confederate Records (Record Group [RG] 109).

CSG   Circulars and Circular Letters, 1861–85 (entry 63), Office of the Surgeon General (Army) (RG 112).

LR   Letters Received, 1818–89 (entry 12), Office of the Surgeon General (Army) (RG 112).

LS   Letters and Endorsements Sent, April 1818–October 1889 (entry 2), Office of the Surgeon General (Army) (RG 112).

LSAL   Letters and Endorsements Sent Relating to Artificial Limbs, Compiled 1864–69 (entry 1395), Records of the U.S. Army Commands, 1817–1947 (RG 393).

LSMO   Letters and Endorsements Sent to Medical Officers, September 1862–September 1872 (entry 7), Office of the Surgeon General (Army) (RG 112).

SSHR   Special Scientific and Historical Records, 1860s–1880s (entry 629), Records of the Adjutant General's Office (RG 94).

1. Melancholy Harvest

1. Hill to C. J. Faulkner, February 25, 1863, *War of the Rebellion*, ser. 1, vol. 12, pt. 2, 669–73; Lenoir to mother, September 13, 1862, Lenoir family papers, personal correspondence, 1861–65, inventory no. 426, Manuscripts Department, Southern Historical Collection, University of North Carolina at Chapel Hill, http://docsouth.unc.edu/imls/lenoir/lenoir.html, accessed April 19, 2010.

2. Baxter, "Charge at Kenesaw."

3. Holmes, "Human Wheel"; *Medical and Surgical History*, pt. 3, vol. 2, ch. 12, 877–80; Bollet, *Civil War Medicine*, 143–60; Bollet, "Amputations in the Civil War."

4. James E. Hanger, "Record of Service" archives of Hanger Orthopedic Group; Little, *Seventh Regiment New Hampshire Volunteers*, 531–35.

5. *Medical and Surgical History*, pt. 3, vol. 2, ch. 12, 877–80.

6. Bollet, *Civil War Medicine*, 143–60; Bollet, "Amputations in the Civil War"; Baxter, "Charge at Kenesaw."

7. *Medical and Surgical History*, pt. 3, vol. 2, ch. 12, 877–80.

8. Gould, *Investigations*, 208–17; McPherson, *For Cause and Comrades*, 181–82; "Palmer's Artificial Limbs."

9. Bagby, "Empty Sleeve."

10. Holmes, "Human Wheel." A discussion of limb technology and how it related to the social needs of amputees appears in Mihm, "A Limb Which Shall Be Presentable."

11. Lenoir to mother, September 13, 1862, Lenoir family papers; Woodward, *Mary Chesnut's Civil War*, 709; Stansbury, *Argument*, 10–11.

12. Hill, *John Smith's Funny Adventures*, 48–54.

13. Lenoir to Thomas J. Lenoir, April 8 and July 23, 1863, Lenoir family papers; Barney, *Making of a Confederate*, 102.

14. Palmer, *Palmer Arm and Leg: Correspondence*, 7; Galloway, "Rev. C. K. Marshall"; W. T. Cole to C. K. Marshall, September 25, 1864, ARMS; Thomas Welch to William A. Carrington, February 17, 1864, file for Welch, Compiled Service Records of Confederate Soldiers Who Served in Organizations from the State of Alabama (microfilm M311, roll 190), RG 109, NARA

15. John M. McKenzie to William A. Hammond, December 15, 1862, LR.

16. Act of July 22, 1861, ch. 9, 12 Stat. 268 (1863); Act of July 14, 1862, ch. 166, 12 Stat. 566 (1863); Act of July 16, 1862, ch. 182, 12 Stat. 582 (1863); Glasson, "History of Military Pension Legislation," 70–87.

17. Carrington, *Brief Review*; Cunningham, *Doctors in Gray*, 144–45; Coddington, "Soldiers' Relief."

18. To date, probably the most detailed account of either program published elsewhere is a brief description of the Confederate effort in McDaid, "How a One-Legged Rebel Lives."

2. The Best Substitutes Known to Art

1. "Claims of Mechanical Surgery"; Selpho, *Best Substitutes*, 16; Palmer, *Palmer Arm and Leg, Adopted*, 41.

2. Selpho, *Best Substitutes*, 7–9; Palmer, "Palmer's Artificial Leg in London"; Potts, "Mr. Potts."

3. Palmer, "Palmer's Artificial Limbs"; Palmer, *Palmer Arm and Leg: Correspondence*, 5; MacDonald, "History of Artificial Limbs"; "B. Frank. Palmer's Portrait." Palmer was inconsistent about the age at which his leg was amputated.

4. Stansbury, *Testimony*.

5. Ibid.; Clement advertisement in Marsh, *Plain and Popular Explanation*, 70–71.

6. The patent count is based on devices listed as "artificial arm and hand," "artificial arm," "artificial hand and arm," "artificial hand," "artificial leg," or "artificial limb" in Leggett, *Subject-Matter Index*. For a discussion about the association between patents and inventive activity for medical devices, see Schmidt, "Multiplicity," 49–52.

7. "Code of Ethics"; Condie, Carpenter, and Ogier, "Apothecaries"; Smith, *Principles and Practice of Surgery*, 716; Hudson, *Artificial Limbs*, 8.

8. George E. Marks, *Treatise on Artificial Limbs*, 17; "Improved Artificial Leg" (1860); "Artificial Legs."

9. Hudson, *Artificial Limbs*, 6–7; "Claims of Mechanical Surgery"; Bly, *New and Important Invention*, 5.

10. Palmer, *Palmer Arm and Leg: Correspondence*; "Medical Intelligence"; Foster, *Brief Description*. Wags joked that the LL.D. sometimes appended to Palmer's name stood for "Leg-um Doctor" ("in the collegiate tongue") or "Lost Leg Department" ("Progress of Medicine," 525).

11. Minor, "Report on Artificial Limbs"; Holmes, "Human Wheel"; Palmer, *Palmer Arm and Leg: Correspondence*, 8.

12. Houston, Bolton, and Joynes, "Report"; George B. Jewett, *Salem Leg*, 3.

13. George E. Marks, *Treatise on Marks' Patent Artificial Limbs*, 10; O. D. Wilcox, Patent 15,831, Artificial Leg, September 30, 1856; J. J. Woodward, Edward Curtis, and

George A. Otis to C. H. Crane, August 13, 1868, SSHR; Kimball and Lawrence to unknown [1864], SSHR.

14. "Artificial Limbs," *New York Times*, March 26, 1855, 1; Clement, *Clement Patent Improved Artificial Leg*, 3; Houston, Bolton, and Joynes, "Report"; B. Frank. Palmer, Patent 22,256, Artificial Arm and Hand, January 11, 1859; Bly, *New and Important Invention*, 5.

15. George E. Marks, *Treatise on Marks' Patent Artificial Limbs*, 18; "Improved Artificial Leg" (1862); George W. Yerger, Patent 7,204, Improvement in Artificial Legs, March 19, 1850; Theodore F. Engelbrecht, Reinhold Boeklen, and William Staehlen, Patent 37,282, Improvement in Artificial Legs, January 6, 1863; Hiram A. Kimball and Andrew J. Lawrence, Patent 54,364, Improvement in Artificial Legs, May 1, 1866; *Monroe and Gardiner's Imperishable Raw Hide Artificial Limbs*; John S. Drake, Patent 9,232, Artificial Leg, August 31, 1852; Robert Murray, John Campbell, and A. K. Smith to William A. Hammond, December 1, 1863, SSHR.

16. George W. Yerger, Patent 7,204, Improvement in Artificial Legs, March 19, 1850; *Transactions of the American Institute for the Year 1850*, 76; "Improved Artificial Leg" (1862).

17. Houston, Bolton, and Joynes, "Report"; Minor, "Report on Artificial Limbs."

18. Selpho, *Best Substitutes*, 11; Bly, *New and Important Invention*, 3; Benjamin W. Jewett, *Jewett's Patent Artificial Leg Company*, 4–5; Minor, "Report on Artificial Limbs"; A. A. Marks, *Marks' Patent Artificial Limbs*.

19. Marvin Lincoln, Patent 39,487, Improvement in Artificial Arms, August 11, 1863; B. Frank. Palmer, Patent 22,576; "Palmer's Artificial Limbs," *Scientific American*; Selpho, *Best Substitutes*; Wales, *Mechanical Therapeutics*, 233; D. W. Kolbe, Patent 45,052, Improvement in Artificial Arms, November 15, 1864.

20. Marvin Lincoln, Patent 39,487, Improvement in Artificial Arms, August 11, 1863; Lincoln, *Lincoln's Patent Artificial Arm*; A. A. Marks, *Marks' Patent Artificial Limbs*, 12–13.

21. Hudson, *Artificial Limbs*, 3, 24–26; Photograph CP 1545, National Museum of Health and Medicine, Washington, D.C.

22. Stansbury, *Testimony*; *Annual Report of the American Institute*, 37; *Transactions of the N.Y. State Agricultural Society*, 281; *Tenth Exhibition*, 89; *Transactions of the American Institute for the Year 1850*, 76; *Transactions of the American Institute for the Year 1857*, 103–4.

23. Freedley, *Philadelphia and Its Manufactures*, 509–10; Matlack to Edwin M. Stanton, December 1, 1862, LR. Palmer's self-promotion and self-congratulation may have peaked in his 112-page booklet *Steps*, which was published in the mid-1870s.

24. Clement, *Clement Patent Improved Artificial Leg*, 1–2; "Artificial Substitutes"; Hudson, *Surgical Adjuvant*.

25. Stansbury, *Argument*, 9; B. Frank. Palmer to W. A. Hammond, October 27, 1862, LR; Palmer, *Palmer Arm and Leg: Correspondence*, 45; Hudson, *Surgical Adjuvant*, 3; "Artificial Substitutes"; "Palmer's Artificial Leg."

26. Selpho advertisement, *New York City Directory, for 1842 and 1843*, 285; Palmer, "Infringements"; Bly, *Nature the Teacher*, 5.

27. Bly, *Nature the Teacher*, 7; Douglass, *Douglass Patent Artificial Limbs*, 5; Palmer, *Palmer Arm and Leg: Correspondence*, 21; Palmer, *Palmer Arm and Leg, Adopted*, 15; Selpho, *Best Substitutes*, 10; Hudson, *Artificial Limbs*, 27; George B. Jewett, *Salem Leg*, 9.

28. Palmer, *Palmer Arm and Leg, Adopted*, 29–31; A. A. Marks, *Marks' Patent Artificial Limbs*, 18; Clement, *Clement Patent Improved Artificial Leg*, 13.

29. Bly, *Nature the Teacher*, 8–9; Selpho, *Best Substitutes*, 25–27; Houston, Bolton, and Joynes, "Report."

30. Carrington, *Brief Review*, 6; Minor, "Report on Artificial Limbs."

3. Noble Charity

1. Satterlee to Hammond, October 9, 1862, SSHR.

2. Act of July 16, 1862, ch. 182, 12 Stat. 582 (1863); Palmer, *Report of the Great National Benefaction*, 1–2; "The Week" (1861); Glasson, "History of Military Pension Legislation," 70–87.

3. Palmer, *Palmer Arm and Leg: Correspondence*, 3–4. The Naval Asylum cared for disabled seamen, naval officers, and marines.

4. Ibid. The Soldiers' Home, also known as the Military Asylum, was the army's counterpart to the Naval Asylum; one of its structures became President Lincoln's "summer White House" in 1862–64 (Goode, *United States Soldiers' Home*).

5. J. R. Smith (for Hammond) to Valentine Mott, August 12, 1862, LS; Act of February 9, 1863, ch. 25, 12 Stat. 642 (1863); Act of March 14, 1864, ch. 30, 13 Stat. 22 (1866); Act of June 15, 1864, ch. 124, 13 Stat. 126 (1866); Appropriations for Furnishing Artificial Limbs and Apparatus or Commutation Thereof (entry 32), Records of the Department of Veterans Affairs (RG 15), NARA; E. S. Dunster (for Hammond) to Satterlee, September 18, 1863, LSMO; Palmer, *Report of the Great National Benefaction*, 4. The amount of money devoted to limbs was relatively small. In the fiscal year ending on June 30, 1862, for example, the army medical and hospital department expended about $2.4 million (Message of the President of the United States, H.R. Exec. Doc. No. 37-1, at 50 [1862]).

6. Gross and Gross, *Autobiography*, 133–34; Satterlee to Hammond, October 9, 1862, SSHR; C. McDougall to Hammond, November 12, 1862, LR.

7. Satterlee to Hammond, October 9, 1862, SSHR.

8. Ibid.; C. H. Alden (for Hammond) to Nichols, September 28, 1862, LS. The Government Hospital for the Insane, which opened in 1855, became a convenient location for the treatment of sick and wounded soldiers and sailors during the war. Some of the military patients began calling the institution St. Elizabeth Hospital, a less pejorative appellation taken from name of the land on which the structures stood (Hurd et al., *Institutional Care of the Insane*, 145–46).

9. Satterlee to Hammond, October 9, 1862, SSHR; Warren to Satterlee, October 8, 1862, SSHR.

10. Gross to Satterlee, October 8, 1862, SSHR.

11. Ibid., Palmer to Gross, October 7, 1862, SSHR.

12. Gross to Satterlee, October 8, 1862, SSHR.

13. J. R. Smith (for Hammond) to C. McDougall, October 13, 1862, LSMO; "Hospitals for the Maimed"; "Maimed Soldiers"; J. R. Smith (for Hammond) to King, October 22, 1862, LSMO; J. R. Smith (for Hammond) to McDougall, November 4, 1862, LSMO.

14. Palmer to Hammond, October 20, 1862, LR.

15. Palmer to Hammond, October 27, 1862, LR; Gross to Hammond, October 23, 1862, LR; McClellan to Hammond, October 24, 1862, LR; Stillé, *History*, 131–32. Palmer told Hammond in his letter of October 27 that he would cease legal proceed-

ings against Jewett and Hudson if the surgeon general so advised. Hammond likely did ask Palmer to stop so as not to interfere with those makers' participation in the limbs program.

16. Selpho to Hammond, October 30, 1862, LR; J. R. Smith (for Hammond) to Selpho, May 7, 1863, LS; J. R. Smith (for Hammond) to Holden, November 8, 1862, LSMO.

17. McDougall to Hammond, October 25, 1862, LR; McDougall to Hammond, November 12, 1862, LR; McDougall to Hammond, November 20, 1862, LR.

18. J. R. Smith (for Hammond) to R. C. Wood, November 14, 1862, LSMO; J. R. Smith (for Hammond) to Wood, December 24, 1862, LSMO; Satterlee to Hammond, October 9, 1862, SSHR.

19. Palmer, *Palmer Arm and Leg: Correspondence*; Stansbury, *Testimony*; E. D. Hudson to C. McDougall, October 28, 1862, LR.

20. Tripler to J. K. Barnes, May 26, 1864, LR; "News from Washington,"*New York Times*, September 25, 1863.

21. McDougall to Hammond, November 20, 1862, LR; J. R. Smith (for Hammond) to McDougall, November 26, 1862, LSMO; J. R. Smith (for Hammond) to William Selpho, May 7, 1863, LS; Tripler to Barnes, May 26, 1864, LR.

22. C. H. Alden (for Hammond) to D. DeForrest Douglas, November 17, 1862, LS.

23. Palmer, *Palmer Arm and Leg: Correspondence*, 8; Satterlee to Hammond, October 9, 1862, SSHR; Bly, *New and Important Invention*, 30; J. R. Smith (for Hammond) to C. McDougall, November 26, 1862, LSMO.

24. "The Week" (1862).

25. Marks to Hammond, October 29, 1862, LR.

26. Douglass to Satterlee, November 13, 1862, LR; C. H. Alden (for Hammond) to Douglass, November 17, 1862, LS; Douglass to Satterlee, November 19, 1862, LR; Douglass advertisement, *Scientific American*, n.s., 7 (November 29, 1862), 351.

27. J. R. Smith (for Hammond) to Douglass, November 15, 1862, LS.

28. Palmer, *Will the American Government*, 6.

29. Matlack to Edwin M. Stanton, December 1, 1862, LR; Gross to Hammond, May 26, 1863, LR; Mott to Hammond, May 25, 1863, LR; Warren to Hammond, March 17, 1863, LR; Fravel to Hammond, December 6, 1862, LR; James E. Yeatman to Hammond, December 4, 1862, LR; J. R. Smith (for Hammond) to Fravel, December 15, 1862, LS; John Neill to John Campbell, 27 March 1865, SSHR.

30. J. R. Smith (for Hammond) to C. McDougall, December 6, 1862, LSMO; E. S. Dunster (for Hammond) to D. L. Magruder, September 21, 1863, LSMO; E. S. Dunster (for Hammond) to George B. Jewett, July 25, 1863, LS; John M. McKenzie to Hammond, December 15, 1862, LR.

31. Bly to Hammond, December 25, 1862, LR; Bly to Hammond, January 22, 1863, LR; Palmer to Charles F. Stansbury, June 1, 1863, LR.

32. Palmer, *Will the American Government*, 2; Palmer, *Palmer Arm and Leg: Correspondence*, 49.

33. "Artificial Limbs," *New York Times*, December 10, 1862; J. K. Barnes, *Artificial Limbs Furnished to Soldiers*, H.R. Exec. Doc. No. 39-108 (1st Sess. 1866). The Barnes report shows, probably in error, three limbs being furnished in 1862 by nonapproved manufacturers and a few being furnished before the program started.

34. J. R. Smith (for Hammond) to Selpho, Bly, Palmer, Hudson, and Jewett, December 31, 1862, LS.

4. Good and Serviceable Limbs

1. R. L. Rea to Hammond, January 6, 1863, LR; J. R. Smith (for Hammond) to J. B. Porter, February 17, 1863, LSMO.

2. J. R. Smith (for Hammond) to McDougall, December 5, 1862, LSMO. No arms had been approved as of late January 1863 (C. C. Byrne [for Hammond] to L. H. Holden, January 24, 1863, LSMO), but an 1866 report shows that eight of the ten arms supplied by Selpho in 1863 were furnished between mid-February and mid-May (J. K. Barnes, Artificial Limbs Furnished to Soldiers, H.R. Exec. Doc. No. 39-108 [1st Sess. 1866]). Two arms furnished in January 1863 may have been among the ones tested in McDougall's patients.

3. E. S. Dunster (for Hammond) to H. A. Gildea, April 29, 1863, LS; E. S. Dunster (for Hammond) to medical directors, May 14, 1863, CSG; E. S. Dunster (for Hammond) to McDougall, May 14, 1863, LSMO; H. A. Gildea to Hammond, June 5, 1863, LR.

4. E. S. Dunster (for Hammond) to medical directors, April 23, 1863, LSMO; William Selpho to Hammond with endorsement by J. H. Puleston, May 5, 1863, LR; Edwin P. Selpho to Hammond, May 9, 1863, LR.

5. J. R. Smith (for Hammond) to William Selpho, May 7, 1863, LS; William Selpho to Hammond, October 30, 1862, LR.

6. J. R. Smith (for Hammond) to J. M. Cuyler, R. Murray, and P. B. Goddard, June 9, 1863, CSG; Palmer, *Will the American Government*, 1–6; Palmer to Charles F. Stansbury, June 1, 1863, LR.

7. C. H. Crane (for J. K. Barnes) to McDougall, October 24, 1863, LSMO; C. H. Crane to Robert Murray, John Campbell, and A. K. Smith, October 6, 1863, LSMO; Murray, Campbell, and Smith to Hammond, December 1, 1863, SSHR; C. H. Crane (for Barnes) to Selpho, December 12, 1863, LS; Palmer, *Palmer Arm and Leg, Adopted*, 11; Palmer, *Will the American Government*, 1.

8. Duncan, "Strange Case of Surgeon General Hammond."

9. B. A. Clements and R. S. Satterlee, Report of a Board of Medical Officers, August 8, 1864, SSHR; C. H. Crane (for Barnes) to medical directors, August 17, 1863, LSMO; W. C. Spencer (for Barnes) to medical directors, August 31, 1863, CSG; Palmer to Board of Surgeons, July 19, 1864, SSHR; Palmer, *Palmer Arm and Leg, Adopted*, 10. The announcement of approvals did not specify whether the approved Bly leg was his ball-and-socket model with lateral ankle movement.

10. Clements and Satterlee, Report of a Board of Medical Officers, August 8, 1864, SSHR.

11. Gildea to E. S. Dunster, December 11, 1863, LR.

12. Clements and Satterlee, Report of a Board of Medical Officers, August 8, 1864, SSHR. Douglass's limbs remained unapproved throughout the war. Douglass's disappointment prompted him to add the following statement to his advertisements starting in March 1866: "No connection whatever with inferior government legs" (*Boston Medical and Surgical Journal* 74 [March 22, 1866], i).

13. Small and McMillen to Barnes, November 29, 1864, SSHR; G. Perin and C. Tripler to Barnes, December 7, 1864, SSHR; W. C. Spencer (for Barnes) to medical directors, December 20, 1864, CSG; John Neill and R. J. Levis to John Campbell, March 27, 1865, SSHR; B. A. Clements and J. Simons, Proceedings of a Board of Medical Officers, May 5, 1865, SSHR.

14. W. C. Spencer (for Barnes) to medical directors, January 23, 1865, CSG.

15. C. H Crane (for Barnes) to W. J. Sloan, H. S. Hewitt, and B. A. Clements, March 1, 1865, CSG; Clements and Simons, Proceedings of a Board of Medical Officers, May 5, 1865, SSHR; C. H. Crane (for Barnes), Circular, May 13, 1865, CSG; C. H. Crane (for Barnes), Memorandum, June 5, 1865, CSG; C. S. Tripler to Barnes, January 16, 1866, SSHR; C. H. Crane (for Barnes), Circular, January 30, 1866, CSG; W. C. Spencer and J. S. Billings to Barnes, May 23, 1866, SSHR; W. C. Spencer (for Barnes), Circular, May 23, 1866, CSG; W. C. Spencer (for Barnes) to medical directors, May 31, 1866, CSG. Hudson had been supplying apparatus for resection at the government's request well before the May 1865 notice of his approval (W. J. Sloan [for C. McDougall] to Hudson, December 14, 1864, LSAL). Edward Spellerberg of Philadelphia supplied enough artificial arms in 1865 to suggest his official approval (J. K. Barnes, Artificial Limbs Furnished to Soldiers, H.R. Exec. Doc. No. 39-108 [1st Sess. 1866]), yet his name appeared on no list of approved makers through that year. It did appear as such, however, in literature of the U.S. Sanitary Commission in 1865 (U.S. Sanitary Commission, *Soldier's Friend*, 38).

16. Bly to Hammond, March 25, 1863, LR; C. H. Alden (for Hammond) to Bly, March 28, 1863, LS.

17. W. J. Sloan (for McDougall) to Theron Shell, March 8, 1864, LSAL; McDougall to William J. Rohrbaugh, October 25, 1864, LSAL; McDougall to Acting Assistant Surgeon Phelps, December 21, 1864, LSAL. Free transportation for limb recipients was not officially authorized by Congress until 1866 (Act of July 28, 1866, ch. 305, 14 Stat. 342 [1868]). How long it usually took for an artificial limb to be provided is unknown. James M. Taylor, formerly of the 96th Illinois Infantry, visited Palmer's office in Philadelphia in March 1865 to be measured for an arm and was told that his prosthesis would be ready in about twenty-five days (James M. Taylor diary, March 29–31, 1865, Taylor family papers, box 1, folder 1, Manuscripts Department, Abraham Lincoln Presidential Library, Springfield, IL). In 1868, Palmer claimed to have 500 artificial limbs in stock and that a customer could be provided with a usable device within hours (Palmer, *Report of the Great National Benefaction*, 34).

18. Palmer to Hammond, April 28, 1863, LR; Act to Provide Internal Revenue to Support the Government and to Pay Interest on the Public Debt, ch. 119, 12 Stat. 432 (1863); *Tax-Payer's Manual*, 1; E. S. Dunster (for Hammond) to Palmer, May 2, 1863, LS; *Laws of the United States Relating to Internal Revenue*, 86.

19. Stanton to John A. Dix, November 24, 1863, *War of the Rebellion*, ser. 2, vol. 7, 69; Entry for Palmer letter P331, March 15, 1864, Registers of Letters Received by the Office of the Secretary of War, Main Series, 1800–1870 (microfilm M22, roll 111), RG 107, NARA; W. Hoffman to Palmer, 22 March 1864, *War of the Rebellion*, ser. 2, vol. 6, 1080.

20. "Crutches for Cripples," (*Placerville, CA*) *Mountain Democrat*, June 4, 1864, 5; Untitled, (*Raleigh*) *North Carolina Standard*, August 10, 1864, 2.

21. Tripler to Barnes, May 26, 1864, LR; Act of July 27, 1868, ch. 264, 15 Stat. 235 (1869); Act of June 30, 1870, ch. 179, 16 Stat. 174 (1871).

22. Selpho to Hammond [May 1863?], LR.

23. Tripler to Barnes, June 20, 1864, LR; A. A. Overman to Morton, May 26, 1864, LR; Sanford B. Hunt (for Tripler) to J. S. Bobbs, June 2, 1864, LR.

24. Fisher to unknown, June 14, 1864, LR; W. C. Spencer (for Barnes) to Tripler, August 13, 1864, LSMO.

25. J. K. Barnes, Report of the Surgeon General, H.R. Exec. Doc. No. 39-1, at 380–81 (2d Sess. 1866).

26. J. K. Barnes, Artificial Limbs Furnished to Soldiers, H.R. Exec. Doc. No. 39-108 (1st Sess. 1866); Welles, *Report of the Secretary*, 148; Barnes, Report of the Surgeon General, H.R. Exec. Doc. No. 39-1, at 380–81 (2d Sess. 1866); *Medical and Surgical History*, pt. 3, vol. 1, 966.

27. Barnes, Artificial Limbs Furnished to Soldiers, H.R. Exec. Doc. No. 39-108 (1st Sess. 1866).

28. Ibid.

29. Palmer, *Report of the Great National Benefaction*; Barnes, Artificial Limbs Furnished to Soldiers, H.R. Exec. Doc. No. 39-108 (1st Sess. 1866); Barnes, Report of the Surgeon General, H.R. Exec. Doc. No. 39-1, at 380–81 (2d Sess. 1866).

30. *Medical and Surgical History*, pt. 3, vol. 2, ch. 12, 877–80; Barnes, Report of the Surgeon General, H.R. Exec. Doc. No. 39-1, at 380–81 (2d Sess. 1866). The estimate of officers accounting for 6 percent of amputees is taken from Union statistics showing that 5.8 percent of the Union killed or wounded were officers (Fox, *Regimental Losses*, 38).

31. Benjamin W. Jewett, *Jewett's Patent Artificial Leg Company*, 2; Barnes, Report of the Surgeon General, H.R. Exec. Doc. No. 39-1, at 380–81 (2d Sess. 1866); Act of June 17, 1870, ch. 132, 16 Stat. 153 (1871).

32. *Medical and Surgical History*, pt. 3, vol. 1, 966.

5. An Act of Esteem and Gratitude

1. "The Meeting for the Relief of Maimed Soldiers," *Richmond Daily Dispatch*, January 27, 1864, 1; Carrington, *Brief Review*, 2–3. The African Church was commonly used by politicians for public meetings (Pollard, *Life of Jefferson Davis*, 469).

2. "Assistance for wounded soldiers," *Richmond Daily Dispatch*, January 16, 1864, 1; Galloway, "Rev. C. K. Marshall"; *Journal of the Congress of the Confederate States of America, 1861–1865*, vol. 6, S. Doc. No. 58-234, at 62 (2d Sess. 1905); Carrington, *Brief Review*, 2.

3. "The Meeting for the Relief of Maimed Soldiers," *Richmond Daily Dispatch*, January 27, 1864, 1. There is no evidence that the abbreviation A.R.M.S. was intended to be pronounced as an acronym. Doing so would have been particularly inappropriate, given the organization's inability to provide artificial arms.

4. Ibid.; File for William A. Carrington, Compiled Service Records of Confederate Generals and Staff Officers, and Nonregimental Enlisted Men (microfilm M331, roll 49), RG 109, NARA; Carrington to Marshall, February 10, 1865, ARMS; James E. Hanger to Carrington, January 16, 1864, ARMS; James L. Cabell to Carrington, January 20, 1864, ARMS.

5. Carrington, *Brief Review*, 2; Carrington to Wells, February 8, 1864, ARMS; Hanger to Carrington, January 16, 1864, ARMS; Wells to Carrington, February 11, 1864, ARMS; James L. Cabell to Carrington, January 20, 1864, ARMS; James E. Hanger, "Record of Service," archives of Hanger Orthopedic Group; "Hanger's L.E.G.," *Staunton (VA) Speculator*, March 10, 1863, 2. Hanger's patents were dated March 23 and August 18, 1863 (Rhodes, *Report of the Commissioner of Patents*, 12); Rufus R. Rhodes to Carrington, January 26, 1864, ARMS). A Union list of prisoners of war showed Hanger as a private in Company D, 23rd Virginia Infantry, but his

name does not appear in the rolls of that or any other Confederate military unit. (H. P. McCain to Commandant, Washington Camp No. 305, Sons of Confederate Veterans, in file for James E. Hanger, Compiled Service Records of Confederate Soldiers Who Served in Organizations from the State of Virginia [microfilm M324, roll 664], RG 109, NARA). Ingraham (*Enabling the Human Spirit*, 41) says Hanger created "the world's first articulated double-joint limb," but prostheses articulated at both the knee and ankle were being made by Potts as early as 1801 and possibly by others before that (Potts, "Mr. Potts"). Ingraham (*Enabling the Human Spirit*, 56) and other sources also state that Hanger moved his shop from Staunton, Virginia, to Richmond during the war, but ARMS correspondence unambiguously places Hanger in Staunton throughout his dealings with that organization (January 1864 through February 1865).

6. Carrington to Smith, January 26, 1864, ARMS; Carrington to Gibson, January 26, 1864, ARMS; John and George Gibson to Carrington, February 6, 1864, ARMS.

7. Carrington to Wells, March 12, 1864, ARMS; Wells to Carrington, March 14, 1864, ARMS.

8. Carrington to Wells, February 8, 1864; Carrington to Rhodes, January 26, 1864, ARMS; Carrington to James L. Cabell, March 1, 1864, ARMS; Carrington to Rhodes, March 1, 1864, ARMS; Carrington to Edward Warren, November 8, 1864, ARMS; Carrington to James Bolton, March 3, 1864, ARMS; Carrington to Spooner and Harris, February 1, 1865, ARMS. It is unclear whether the Bly model admired by Carrington was the one with lateral ankle motion.

9. For a thorough description of Dahlgren's raid and the controversy concerning his papers, see Wittenberg, *Like a Meteor Blazing Brightly*.

10. Ibid.; Carrington to Seddon, March 7, 1864, ARMS; Carrington to Lee, March 12, 1864, ARMS; Lee, "Death of Colonel Dahlgren"; Carrington to Wells, March 12, 1864, ARMS; Wells to Carrington, May 5, 1864, ARMS; Schultz, *Dahlgren Affair*, 259; Williamson, *Mosby's Rangers*, 79; Dahlgren, *Memoir of Ulric Dahlgren*, 276.

11. Carrington to Sims, March 19, 1864, ARMS; Carrington to Edward Warren, November 8, 1864, ARMS.

12. Ewell to Wells, February 24, 1864, ARMS; Hancock to Carrington, February 29, 1864, ARMS. In November 1865, Ewell provided a similar testimonial for a newly acquired Northern leg. According to the maker, Richard Clement, Ewell "wore an inferior substitute [presumably the Wells leg] till the time he was fitted by me" (Clement, *Clement Patent Improved Artificial Leg*, 5).

13. Confederate States, Adjutant and Inspector General's Office (AIGO), special orders no. 279, November 24, 1863, paragraph 15; "Hood's Legs," *Richmond Daily Dispatch*, January 14, 1865, 3. The newspaper account referred to Darby but did not name him. It identified Hood's leg as an Anglesey model, which was made by Gray.

14. Letter registry entry (D434) for Darby to Adjutant and Inspector General's Office, April 18, 1864, Register of Letters Received (vol. 63), Records of the Adjutant and Inspector General's Office (ch. 1), War Department Collection of Confederate Records (R G 109), NARA; Carrington to Darby, October 14, 1864, ARMS; Darby to Carrington, November 9, 1864, ARMS. Although Darby stated that Hood had never used a French leg, other accounts say that he did (Woodward, *Mary Chesnut's Civil War*, 709; Custer, *Tenting on the Plain*, 37–38).

15. Butler to Carrington, December 14, 1864, ARMS; Carrington to Walker, December 22, 1864, ARMS; G. T. Beauregard to S. Cooper, *War of the Rebellion*, ser. 1, vol. 36, pt. 3, 841; Walker to S. Cooper, September 24, 1864, ARMS; Walker to Carrington, January 3, 1865, ARMS; Diary of Dr. David Warman, private collection.

16. Carrington to Cabell and Davis, February 10, 1864, ARMS; Carrington, *Brief Review*, 6; Cabell to Carrington, February 12, 1864, ARMS. The third Confederate patent for an artificial leg was granted to Wells and Brother on August 11, 1864 (Rhodes, *Annual Report of the Commissioner of Patents*, 6).

17. Carrington, *Brief Review*, 6–7; Hanger to Carrington, January 16, 1864, ARMS; Hanger to Carrington, February 16, 1864, ARMS; Carrington to Hay and Merillat, March 12, 1864, ARMS; Hay to Carrington, March 22, 1864, ARMS. It is puzzling that Hanger would use steel in a modification of the Palmer limb, which was made of willow.

18. Carrington to James A. Seddon, March 1, 1864, ARMS; Hanger to Carrington, February 16, 1864, ARMS; Wells and Brother to Carrington, March 14, 1864, ARMS; Carrington, "Artificial Limbs—How to Make Them," 59.

19. Mayo to Carrington, May 23, 1864, ARMS; AIGO, special orders no. 217, September 13, 1864, paragraph 2; Carrington to Mayo, October 14, 1864, ARMS; Carrington, Report of the Corresponding Secretary, May 2, 1864, ARMS; AIGO, special orders no. 272, November 20, 1862, paragraph 21.

20. Davis to Carrington, March 1, 1864, ARMS. Carrington referred to Davis holding a patent—presumably for an artificial limb—but none appears among United States or Confederate patent records (Carrington to Davis, February 26, 1864, ARMS). Levi G. Davis, p. 20, line 1, free inhabitants of Fluvanna County, Virginia Census of Population, Eighth Census of the U.S. (microfilm M653, roll 944), RG 29, NARA; Hodgson to George A. Trenholm, file for Hodgson, Confederate Papers Relating to Citizens and Business Firms (microfilm M346, roll 453), RG 109, NARA. Carrington, Report of the Corresponding Secretary, October 10, 1864, ARMS. Strasser was granted on August 16, 1864, the fourth and final patent for an artificial limb recorded in Confederate Patent Office reports (Rhodes, *Annual Report of the Commissioner of Patents*, 6). Cole to Charles K. Marshall, September 25, 1864, ARMS; Spooner to Carrington, November 25, 1864, ARMS; Dolan to Carrington, November 25, 1864, ARMS.

21. Carrington, *Brief Report*, 4; Carrington to Cole, October 24, 1864, ARMS; Carrington, Report of the Corresponding Secretary, n.d., ARMS; Carrington to Cole, December 5, 1864, ARMS; Carrington to Strasser and Callahan, December 5, 1864; Carrington to Charles K. Marshall, January 23, 1865, ARMS; Carrington to Marshall, February 10, 1865, ARMS; Carrington, *Brief Review*, 6–7; Register of orders for artificial limbs, ARMS.

22. Hay to Carrington, March 22, 1864, ARMS; Carrington to Hanger, March 28, 1864; ARMS application for limb, file for Daingerfield, Compiled Service Records of Confederate Soldiers Who Served in Organizations from the State of Virginia (microfilm M324, roll 111), RG 109, NARA. Like Hanger, Daingerfield seemed to have a legitimate claim to being the first amputee of the war.

23. Carrington to Fauntleroy, January 5, 1865, ARMS.

24. Fauntleroy to Carrington, January 10, 1865, ARMS.

25. Carrington to James L. Cabell, January 22, 1864; Carrington to Wells and Brother, December 9, 1864; Carrington to Marshall, January 23, 1865; Carrington to Wells and Brother, December 22, 1864.

26. Cabell to Carrington, February 24, 1864, ARMS; Carrington to Cabell, March 3, 1864, ARMS; Carrington to Taylor, March 13, 1864, ARMS; Carrington to Taylor, September 23, 1864, ARMS; Taylor to Carrington, March 4, 1864, ARMS; Carrington to Hanger, March 19, 1864, ARMS; Hanger to Carrington, September 7, 1864, ARMS; Carrington to Cone, March 3, 1864.

27. Carrington to Bradley, November 29, 1864, ARMS; Carrington to Bradley, December 22, 1864, ARMS.

28. Carrington, *Brief Review*, 2; Thomas D. Bell to Carrington, n.d., ARMS; Carrington to Bell, April 11, 1864; Carrington to James B. Ferguson, February 7, 1864, ARMS.

29. Carrington, *Brief Review*, 2-3.

6. Manifold Difficulties

1. For the difficulties facing Confederate manufacturers, see Wilson, *Confederate Industry*.

2. Moore, *Conscription and Conflict in the Confederacy*; Carrington to Wells, February 10, 1864, ARMS.

3. Wells to Carrington, March 14, 1864, ARMS; Carrington to Wells, March 19, 1864; Hanger to Carrington, September 7, 1864, ARMS; Dolan to Carrington, November 25, 1864, ARMS; Wells to Carrington, December 7, 1864, ARMS.

4. File for John M. Hanger, Compiled Service Records of Confederate Soldiers Who Served in Organizations from the State of Virginia (microfilm M324, roll 423), RG 109, NARA; Hanger to Carrington, October 29, 1864, ARMS.

5. Cabell to Carrington, February 21, 1865, ARMS. Although one researcher has said that ARMS operated the Soldier's Home Hospital in Richmond (Calcutt, *Richmond's Wartime Hospitals*, 177-78), the records of ARMS do not so indicate. The only thing ARMS and that hospital seem to have had in common was the book in which some of their records were kept.

6. File for William Engleheart, Compiled Service Records of Confederate Soldiers Who Served in Organizations from the State of Alabama (microfilm M311, roll 5), RG 109, NARA.

7. Carrington to Wells, March 12, 1864, ARMS; Wells to Carrington, March 14, 1865; Hanger to Carrington, February 16, 1864, ARMS; Carrington to Sims, March 19, 1864, ARMS.

8. Wells to Carrington, August 28, 1864; Hanger to Carrington, January 1, 1865, file for Hanger and Brother, Confederate Papers Relating to Citizens or Business Firms (microfilm M346, roll 401), RG 109, NARA; Weidenmier, "Turning Points."

9. Bee to Carrington, September 23, 1864; ARMS; Carrington, Report of the Corresponding Secretary, October 10, 1864, ARMS; Bee to Carrington, September 26, 1864, ARMS; Carrington to Bee, October 25, 1864, ARMS; Carrington, Report of the Corresponding Secretary, n.d., ARMS; Carrington to Bee, October 29, 1864, ARMS; Carrington, *Brief Review*, 4. For Bee's and Trenholm's involvement in blockade running, see Wise, *Lifeline of the Confederacy*.

10. Carrington to James B. Ferguson, February 7, 1865, ARMS.

11. Carrington to Alexander R. Lawton, December 22, 1864, ARMS; Carrington to Hanger, January 5, 1865, ARMS; Wells to Carrington, January 11, 1865, ARMS; Carrington to Hanger, January 14, 1865, ARMS; Carrington to Frederick W. Sims, January 8, 1865, ARMS; Richard Morton to Carrington, January 12, 1865, ARMS; Carrington to Wells, January 15, 1865, Carrington to Wells, February 27, 1865, ARMS.

12. Hanger to Carrington, December 4, 1864, ARMS; Carrington to John B. Baldwin, December 22, 1864; Carrington to Wells, February 27, 1865; ARMS. Stringent tax laws were enacted in the Confederacy on April 24, 1863, and February 17, 1864 (Schwab, *Confederate States of America*, 284–312; *Laws of Congress*).

13. Carrington, *Brief Review*, 2–5; Carrington to Wells, Hanger, William T. Cole, Strasser and Callahan, and D. W. Hughes and Co., December 5, 1864, ARMS; Carrington to Spooner and Harris, December 22, 1864, ARMS.

14. Treasurer's accounts and finances, ARMS; Carrington, *Brief Review*, 3–4.

15. Carrington to Forrest, February 7, 1865, ARMS; "The Black Flag: Horrible Massacre by Rebels," *New York Times*, April 16, 1864, 1. Carrington referred to the donation coming from citizens of Mississippi rather than Alabama.

16. "General Forrest and the Negroes," *Richmond Daily Dispatch*, August 20, 1864, 1. Some Southern blacks evidently feared Northerners and may well have thought of Forrest as their protector. "Our negroes," wrote one Virginian, "will fight you all [Northerners] nearly as unanimous as their masters; for they, too, know the meanets [*sic*] masters in the South are Yankees who have settled among us" (Whitson, "Letters from the South").

17. Stephens to Carrington, February 20, 1864, ARMS; Carrington to Stephens, March 10, 1864, ARMS.

18. Carrington to Charles Minnegerode, March 15, 1864, ARMS; Carrington, *Brief Review*, 3; Carrington to Charles K. Marshall, January 23, 1865, ARMS; Carrington to Stirewalt, March 19, 1864; ARMS; Stirewalt to Charles Minnegerode, January 30, 1865, ARMS; William N. Nelson to Carrington, February 2, 1865, ARMS.

19. Neely to Carrington, March 9, 1864, ARMS; Carrington, *Brief Review*, 3.

20. Carrington to Seddon, March 1, 1864, ARMS.

21. Warren to Carrington, September 24, 1864, ARMS; Warren, *Report of the Surgeon General of North Carolina*, 20; Carrington to Vance, March 13, 1865, ARMS; Carrington to Murrah, October 27, 1864, ARMS; Lubbock to Murrah, November 1, 1864, ARMS; John Perkins to Charles K. Marshall, February 4, 1865, ARMS; Carrington to Charles K. Marshall, February 10, 1865, ARMS.

22. Carrington to Ferguson, February 7, 1865, ARMS; "The 'Southern Bazaar' in Liverpool: Raising Funds for the Rebels," *New York Times*, November 3, 1864, 1; "British Impertinence Fitly Rebuked," *New York Times*, December 10, 1864, 4; Wharncliffe to Adams, November 12, 1864, *Papers Relating to Foreign Affairs (1865)*, 354–55; Officer, "Dollar-Pound Exchange Rate"; Seward to Adams, December 5, 1864, *Papers Relating to Foreign Affairs (1865)*, 367–68; Adams to Wharncliffe, December 20, 1864, *Papers Relating to Foreign Affairs (1866)*, 61; "Wednesday Morning," *Richmond Daily Dispatch*, December 14, 1864, 2.

23. Carrington to William C. Bee, December 16, 1864, ARMS; Carrington to Wharncliffe, February 7, 1865, ARMS.

24. Carrington, *Brief Review*, 9; Carrington, Report of the Corresponding Secretary, October 10, 1864, ARMS; James L. Cabell to Carrington, January 24, 1865, ARMS; Carrington to Archibald N. Fauntleroy, January 26, 1865.

25. Carrington to Wells, December 5, 1864, ARMS; Wells to Carrington, December 7, 1864, ARMS; Hanger to Carrington, January 1, 1865, file for Hanger and Brother, Confederate Papers Relating to Citizens or Business Firms (microfilm M346, roll 401), RG 109, NARA; Carrington to Archibald N. Fauntleroy, January 5, 1865, ARMS; Charles K. Marshall to Carrington, March 12, 1864, ARMS.

26. Carrington, Report of the Corresponding Secretary, May 2, 1864, ARMS.

27. Carrington to Bee, October 25, 1864, ARMS; Carrington to Pendleton Murrah, October 27, 1864, ARMS; Register of orders for artificial legs, ARMS; Carrington, Report of the Corresponding Secretary, October 10, 1864, ARMS; Carrington to Louis T. Wigfall and Alexander R. Holladay, March 6, 1865, ARMS.

28. Treasurer's accounts and finances, ARMS; Carrington, *Brief Review*, 3; Carrington to Thomas D. Bell, March 15, 1865, ARMS.

29. Carrington to William C. Bee, January 23, 1865, ARMS; Carrington, Report of the Corresponding Secretary, May 2, 1864, ARMS;

30. Carrington to Marshall, February 10, 1865, ARMS;

31. Carrington, *Brief Review*, 4; Treasurer's accounts and finances, ARMS.

32. Carrington to Wigfall and Holladay, March 6, 1865, ARMS; "Proceedings of the Second Confederate Congress," 450–61; *Journal of the Congress of the Confederate States of America, 1861–1865*, vol. 4, S. Doc. No. 58-234, at 712 (2d Sess. 1904).

33. Dyer, *Compendium*, 960; Treasurer's accounts and finances, ARMS.

34. Register of orders for artificial legs, ARMS. Orders in the register were numbered up to 769, but one number was stricken, one omitted, and one used twice. There were also twenty-three duplicate and two triplicate orders for the same applicants.

35. Carrington, Report of the Corresponding Secretary, October 10, 1864, ARMS.

7. Magnificent Benefaction

1. "Artificial Limb," *Southern Confederacy (Atlanta)*, December 28, 1862, 1.

2. Levi G. Davis, free inhabitants of Fluvanna County, Virginia, Census of Population, Eighth Census of the U.S. (microfilm M653, roll 944), p. 20, line 1, RG 29, NARA; Thomas R. Dolan to William A. Carrington, November 25, 1864, ARMS.

3. Edmonson, *American Surgical Instruments*, 54–60.

4. Houston, Bolton, and Joynes, "Report."

5. Gildea advertisement, *Richmond Medical Journal* 1 (1866 May); Palmer advertisement, *Richmond Medical Journal* 1 (1866 June); Clement, *Clement Patent Improved Artificial Leg*, 4–13.

6. Palmer advertisement, *Southern Journal of the Medical Sciences* 1 (1866); Benjamin W. Jewett, *Jewett's Patent Artificial Leg Company*; Hudson advertisement, *Richmond Medical Journal* 1 (January 1866); Bly advertisement, *Southern Journal of the Medical Sciences* 1 (1866); Bly advertisement, *Charleston (SC) Daily News*, 29 December 29, 1866, 3.

7. *Columbia (SC) Daily Phoenix*, July 28, 1865, 2; National Leg and Arm Company advertisement, *Scott's Monthly Magazine* 1 (January 1866): 441; "Southern Manufactures," *Columbia (SC) Daily Phoenix*, May 27, 1866, 2; Southern Leg and Arm Company advertisement, *Columbia (SC) Daily Phoenix*, May 27, 1866, 3; Harvey L. Byrd, Patent 52,964, Improvement in Artificial Legs, March 6, 1866; Houston, Bolton, and Joynes, "Report," 566. When Byrd submitted his limb in 1868 for approval by the Union program, the panel of army surgeons declared that the purported advantages

of the limb were "completely illusory" (Joseph Janvier Woodward, Edward Curtis, and George A. Otis to Surgeon General's Office, August 13, 1868, SSHR).

8. Glasson, "South's Pension and Relief Provisions"; Wegner, *Phantom Pain*, 19–33, 236–37; Res. of Jan. 23 and Mar. 12, 1866, 1866 Gen. Assemb., Spec. Sess. (N.C. 1866); Gen. Assemb. Legis. Doc. No. 11, 1866–67 Sess. (N.C. 1867).

9. McDaid, "How a One-Legged Rebel Lives"; Orr, *Message No. 1*, 25–26; McCawley, *Artificial Limbs*; Candler, *Confederate Records*, 523, 534–38, 578–80, 594–95. An advertisement for Bly (*Charleston [SC] Daily News*, December 29, 1866, 3) indicated that Bly also had the Tennessee state contract.

10. Gen. Assemb. Act No. 643, 1866–67 Sess. (Ala. 1867); Gen. Assemb. Act No. 31, 1866–67 Sess. (Ark. 1867); Gen. Assemb. Act Ch. 1545 (No. 12), 14th Gen. Assemb., 2d Sess. (Fla. 1867); Confederated Southern Memorial Association, *History*, 171; Porter, Circular; Roberts, *Nashville and Her Trade*, 175; Gen. Assemb. Act No. 69, 1880 Sess. (La. 1880); Wegner, *Phantom Pain*, 33–34.

11. Act of June 17, 1870, ch. 132, 16 Stat. 153 (1871); Act of June 8, 1872, ch. 353, 17 Stat. 338 (1873); Act of August 15, 1876, ch. 300, 19 Stat. 203 (1877); Act of March 3, 1891, ch. 562, 26 Stat. 1103 (1891); Report (to accompany H.R. 949), S. Rep. No. 51–4291 (1891); Marks, *Manual*, 241.

12. Sutherland, *Report*, 7–11.

13. Report of the Secretary of War, H.R. Exec. Doc. No. 42-1, pt. 2, at 238 (1871); Sutherland, *Report*, 7–11.

14. Taylor, *Annual Report*, 12; Taylor, *Report*, 15; Bell, *Annual Report*, 48.

15. Sutherland, *Report*, 7–11; Winthrop, *Digest of Opinions*, 575–76.

16. Advertisements, *Station Agent* 9 (March 1893); "Cripples with Improved Feet: More Maiming Done by Railway Cars and Machinery Than by Wars," *New York Sun*, December 3, 1882, 3; Ott, "Sum of Its Parts," 26; George E. Marks, *Treatise* (1888), 159; Winkley Orthotics and Prosthetics, http://www.winkley.com/Pages/NaviPages/History%20Timeline.htm, accessed February 23, 2011; Hanger Orthopedic Group, Press Release, February 9, 2011. In an 1892 advertisement, Winkley touted itself as the "largest firm (excepting one) in the U.S." (*Locomotive Firemen's Magazine* [April 1892], 371).

17. U.S. Sanitary Commission, *Soldier's Friend*, 36–38; Lewis, *Report of the General Superintendent*, 19–20; Stillé, *History*; Bellows, *Provision Required*.

18. Resnick, Gambel, and Hawk, "Historical Perspectives"; Pasquina et al., "Introduction."

19. Carrington, *Brief Review*, 2.

Appendix A. Makers and Inventors Associated with the Union and Confederate Artificial-Limbs Programs

1. Bliss to C. S. Tripler, 13 January 1866, SSHR; "Obituary: D. Willard Bliss"; G. A. Otis and J. S. Billings, Report of Proceedings of a Board of Surgeons, December 18, 1865, SSHR; C. H. Crane (for J. K. Barnes), Circular, January 30, 1866, CSG; Houston, Bolton, and Joynes, "Report." An entry for the company in a city directory indicates a patent date that matches that of Walber's patent (*Boyd's Directory*, 22).

2. Carrington, *Brief Review*, 6.

3. Ibid.

4. Houston, Bolton, and Joynes, "Report."

5. R. Murray, J. Campbell, and A. K. Smith to W. A. Hammond, December 1, 1863, SSHR.

6. R. S. Satterlee to Hammond, October 9, 1862, SSHR; B. A. Clements and J. Simons, Proceedings of a Board of Medical Officers, May 5, 1865, SSHR.

7. An advertisement by Weston (*Harper's Weekly*, February 21, 1863) indicated a patent date that applied to Engelbrecht's patent.

8. Foster, *Brief Description*; Clements and Satterlee, Report of a Board of Medical Officers, August 8, 1864, SSHR.

9. Grenell to Board of Examiners, July 25, 1864, SSHR. Although most published sources give Grenell's initials as J. M., an advertisement in a city directory showed him as I. M. Grenell, and his personal listing showed him as Increase M. Grenell (*Trow's* [1866], 3, 385).

10. Clements and Simons, Proceedings of a Board of Medical Officers, May 5, 1865, SSHR.

11. Carrington, *Brief Review*, 6.

12. *Obituary Record*, 41–42.

13. Leacock advertisement, *Richmond Medical Journal* 1 (June 1866). Houston, Bolton, and Joynes, "Report."

14. Stansbury, *Testimony*, 41–43; Lincoln, *Lincoln's Patent Artificial Arm.*

15. Clements and Simons, Proceedings of a Board of Medical Officers, May 5, 1865, SSHR.

16. A. A. Marks, *Marks' Patent Artificial Limbs*; George E. Marks, *Treatise on Artificial Limbs*, iv; 11.

17. W. H. Miller to Board of Medical Officers, 1864, SSHR.

18. Murray, Campbell, and Smith to Hammond, December 1, 1863, SSHR.

19. Clements and Simons, Proceedings of a Board of Medical Officers, May 5, 1865, SSHR.

20. *Wilson's New York City Copartnership Directory*, 37; *New York City Directory* [1868?], commercial register, 3; *Trow's* (1865), 27; W. J. Sloan to J. K. Barnes, June 14, 1866, SSHR. The firm's name often appears incorrectly as the National Arm and Leg Company.

21. Palmer, *Report of the Great National Benefaction*, 33.

22. Clements and Simons, Proceedings of a Board of Medical Officers, May 5, 1865, SSHR.

23. Ibid.

24. Houston, Bolton, and Joynes, "Report."

25. Clements and Simons, Proceedings of a Board of Medical Officers, May 5, 1865, SSHR.

26. Ibid.

27. C. K. Marshall to Carrington, March 12, 1864, ARMS; Carrington, ARMS minutes, n.d., ARMS.

28. Small and McMillen, *American Leg*; Clements and Simons, Proceedings of a Board of Medical Officers, 5 May 1865, SSHR. McMillen's full name has not been determined. The 1866 list of Union limb recipients indicates that the company was based in Indianapolis (J. K. Barnes, Artificial Limbs Furnished to Soldiers, H.R. Exec. Doc. No. 39-108 [1st Sess. 1866]).

29. Houston, Bolton, and Joynes, "Report." The company often appears as the Southern Arm and Leg Company.

30. Clements and Simons, Proceedings of a Board of Medical Officers, May 5, 1865, SSHR; E. Bentley, R. B. Bontecou, and H. Allen, Proceedings of a Board of Medical Officers, October 26, 1865, SSHR.

31. Carrington, Report of the Corresponding Secretary, October 1864, ARMS.

32. Clements and Simons, Proceedings of a Board of Medical Officers, May 5, 1865, SSHR.

33. Wells and Walber to Satterlee, McDougall, and Clements, 1864, SSHR; Clements and Satterlee, Report of a Board of Medical Officers, August 8, 1864, SSHR.

34. Ibid.; Murray, Campbell, and Smith to Hammond, December 1, 1863, SSHR.

35. Weston to Board of Medical Officers, July 21, 1864, SSHR; Clements and Simons, Proceedings of a Board of Medical Officers, May 5, 1865, SSHR.

Appendix B. Artificial Limbs and Resection Apparatus Supplied to U.S. Soldiers and Sailors by May 10, 1866

1. C. H. Alden (for W. A. Hammond) to C. H. Nichols, September 28, 1862, LS.

2. J. R. Smith (for Hammond) to W. S. King, October 22, 1862, LSMO.

3. Includes one leg reported to have been supplied in 1861.

4. C. McDougall to Hammond, November 12, 1862, LR.

5. J. R. Smith (for Hammond) to R. C. Wood, November 14, 1862, LSMO.

6. Ibid. Selpho's initial approval was revoked in April 1863. E. S. Dunster (for Hammond) to medical directors, April 23, 1863, LSMO.

7. C. H. Crane (for J. K. Barnes) to medical directors, August 17, 1864, LSMO.

8. J. R. Smith (for Hammond) to J. B. Porter, February 17, 1863, LSMO.

9. W. C. Spencer (for Barnes) to medical directors, December 20, 1864, CSG.

10. C. H. Crane (for Barnes) to medical directors, May 13, 1865, CSG.

11. Includes limbs from companies not known to have been approved leg or foot suppliers: P. Daniels, I. M. Grenell, D. W. Kolbe, M. Lincoln, National Leg and Arm Company, and J. W. Weston.

12. C. C. Byron (for Hammond) to S. H. Holden, January 24, 1863, LSMO; J. Bryson to Hammond, May 10, 1863, LR. Selpho's initial approval was revoked in April 1863.

13. C. H. Crane (for Barnes) to W. Selpho et al., December 12, 1863, LS.

14. E. S. Dunster (for Hammond) to J. Bryson, May 14, 1863, LS.

15. W. C. Spencer (for Barnes) to medical directors, January 23, 1865, CSG.

16. Three fingers supplied to one soldier are counted as one hand.

17. W. C. Spencer (for Barnes) to medical directors, May 31, 1866, CSG.

18. Includes limbs from companies not known to have been approved arm or hand suppliers: D. Bly, E. D. Hudson, B. W. Jewett, and Salem Leg Company.

19. W. J. Sloan (for C. McDougall) to E. D. Hudson, December 14, 1864, LSAL.

20. Includes devices from companies not known to have been approved apparatus suppliers: J. H. Gemrig, H. A. Gildea, and M. Lincoln.

BIBLIOGRAPHY

Archives

Austin, Tex.
> Hanger Orthopedic Group

Bethesda, Md.
> National Library of Medicine, History of Medicine Division
> > Images from the History of Medicine

Chapel Hill, N.C.
> University of North Carolina, Southern Historical Collection
> > Lenoir Family Papers

Frederick, Md.
> National Museum of Civil War Medicine

Springfield, Ill.
> Abraham Lincoln Presidential Library
> > James M. Taylor Family Papers

Washington, D.C.
> National Archives and Records Administration
> > RG 15: Records of the Department of Veterans Affairs, 1773–2007
> > RG 29: Records of the Bureau of the Census
> > RG 94: Records of the Adjutant General's Office
> > RG 107: Records of the Office of the Secretary of War
> > RG 109: War Department Collection of Confederate Records
> > RG 112: Office of the Surgeon General (Army)
> > RG 393: Records of U.S. Army Commands, 1817–1947
> National Museum of Health and Medicine

Printed and Online Material

Annual Report of the American Institute, of the City of New-York, for the Years 1863, '64. Albany, N.Y.: Comstock & Cassidy, 1864.

"Artificial Legs." *People's Dental Journal* 1 (July 1863): 74.

"Artificial Substitutes for Lost Legs." *College Journal of Medical Science* 4 (January 1859): 48.

Bagby, J. R. "The Empty Sleeve." In *War Poetry of the South*, edited by William Gilmore Simms, 346–49. New York: Richardson & Co., 1867.

Barney, William T. *The Making of a Confederate: Walter Lenoir's Civil War.* New York: Oxford University Press, 2008.

Baxter, W. H. "The Charge at Kenesaw, and Other Items." In *Every-Day Soldier Life; or A History of the One Hundred and Thirteenth Ohio Volunteer Infantry*, by F. M. McAdams, 341–48. Columbus, Ohio: Charles M Cott & Co., 1884.

Bell, T. F. Annual Report of the Adjutant General of the State of Louisiana for the Year Ending December 31, 1893. Baton Rouge: Advocate, 1894.

Bellows, Henry W. *Provision Required for the Relief and Support of Disabled Soldiers and Sailors and Their Dependents.* Doc. no. 95. New York: U.S. Sanitary Commission, 1866.

"B. Frank. Palmer's Portrait." *Scalpel* 23 (May 1854): 448–49.

Bly, Douglas. *Nature the Teacher—Man the Scholar! And a New, Curious, and Important Invention: The Result.* New York, 1861.

———. *A New and Important Invention.* Rochester, N.Y.: Curtis, Butts & Co., 1862.

Bollet, Alfred Jay. "Amputations in the Civil War." In *Years of Change and Suffering: Modern Perspectives on Civil War Medicine,* edited by James R. Schmidt and Guy R. Hasegawa, 57–67. Roseville, Minn.: Edinborough, 2009.

———. *Civil War Medicine: Challenges and Triumphs.* Tucson: Galen Press, 2002.

Boyd's Directory of Washington and Georgetown. Washington, D.C.: William W. Boyd, 1869.

Calcutt, Rebecca Barbour. *Richmond's Wartime Hospitals.* Gretna, La.: Pelican, 2005.

Candler, Allen D. *The Confederate Records of the State of Georgia,* vol. 4. Atlanta: Chas. P. Byrd, 1910.

Carrington, William A. "Artificial Limbs—How to Make Them." *Confederate States Medical and Surgical Journal* 1 (April 1864): 59.

———. *Brief Review of the Plan and Operations of the Association for the Relief of Maimed Soldiers.* Richmond: ARMS, 1865.

"Claims of Mechanical Surgery." *American Medical Times* 4 (10 May 1862): 267–7.

Clement, Richard. *The Clement Patent Improved Artificial Leg, Adopted for the U.S. Army and Navy, by the Surgeon-Gen'l U.S.A.* Philadelphia: Samuel Loag, 1868.

Coddington, Edward B. "Soldiers' Relief in the Seaboard States of the Southern Confederacy." *Mississippi Valley Historical Review* 37 (June 1950): 17–38.

"Code of Ethics of the American Medical Association, Adopted May, 1847." In *Transactions of the American Medical Association,* 15:355–68. Philadelphia: Collins, 1865.

Condie, D. Francis, James S. Carpenter, and Sept. A. Ogier. "Apothecaries—Patent and Quack Medicines." *American Medical Gazette and Journal of Health* 7 (August 1856): 481–86.

Confederated Southern Memorial Association. *History of the Confederated Memorial Associations of the South.* New Orleans: Graham, 1904.

Cunningham H. H. *Doctors in Gray: The Confederate Medical Service.* Baton Rouge: Louisiana State University Press, 1958.

Custer, Elizabeth B. *Tenting on the Plain; or, General Custer in Kansas and Texas.* New York: Harper & Brothers, 1895.

Dahlgren, John A. *Memoir of Ulric Dahlgren.* Philadelphia: Lippincott, 1872.

Douglass, D. DeForrest. *The Douglass Patent Artificial Limbs,* 8th ed. Springfield, Mass.: Samuel Bowles, 1865.

Duncan, Louis C. "The Strange Case of Surgeon General Hammond," pts. 1 and 2. *Military Surgeon* 64 (January 1929): 98–110; 64 (February 1929): 252–62.

Dyer, Frederick H. *A Compendium of the War of the Rebellion,* pt. 2. De Moines: Dyer, 1908.

Edmonson, James M. *American Surgical Instruments: An Illustrated History of Their Manufacture and a Directory of Instrument Makers to 1900.* San Francisco: Norman, 1997.

Foster, James A. *A Brief Description of James A. Foster's Patent Union Artificial Limbs.* N.p. [1868?].

Fox, William F. *Regimental Losses in the American Civil War, 1861–1865.* Albany, N.Y.: Albany, 1889.

Freedley, Edwin T. *Philadelphia and Its Manufactures: A Hand-Book of the Great Manufactories and Representative Mercantile Houses of Philadelphia, in 1867.* Philadelphia: Edward Young, 1867.

Galloway, Charles B. "The Rev. C. K. Marshall, D.D." *Methodist Quarterly Review* 10 (July 1891): 375–94.

Glasson, William Henry. "History of Military Pension Legislation in the United States." Ph.D. diss., Columbia University, 1900.

———. "The South's Pension and Relief Provision for the Soldiers of the Confederacy." In *Proceedings of the Eighteenth Annual Session of the State Literary and Historical Association of North Carolina*, 61–71. Raleigh: Edwards & Broughton, 1918.

Goode, Paul R. *The United States Soldiers' Home: A History of its First Hundred Years.* Richmond: William Byrd, 1957.

Gould, Benjamin Arthorp. *Investigations in the Military and Anthropological Statistics of American Soldiers.* New York: Hurd and Houghton, 1869.

Gross, Samuel W., and A. Haller Gross, eds. *Autobiography of Samuel D. Gross, M.D.* Philadelphia: George Barrie, 1887.

Hill, A. F. *John Smith's Funny Adventures on a Crutch; or, The Remarkable Peregrinations of a One-Legged Soldier after the War.* Philadelphia: John E. Potter, 1869.

Holmes, Oliver Wendell. "The Human Wheel, Its Spokes and Felloes." *Atlantic Monthly*, May 1863, 567–80.

"Hospitals for the Maimed." *Medical and Surgical Reporter*, n.s., 9 (November 22, 1862): 202.

Houston, M. H., J. Bolton, and L. S. Joynes. "Report of the Richmond Medical Journal Commission." *Richmond Medical Journal* 1 (June 1866): 564–72.

Hudson, E. D. *Artificial Limbs for the United States Army and Navy.* New York [1865?].

———. *The Surgical Adjuvant Remedial.* New York [1864?].

Hurd, Henry M., William F. Drewry, Richard Dewey, Charles W. Pilgrim, G. Alter Blumer, and T. J. W. Burgess. *The Institutional Care of the Insane in the United States and Canada*, vol. 2. Baltimore: Johns Hopkins Press, 1916.

"Improved Artificial Leg." *Scientific American*, April 7, 1860, 240.

"Improved Artificial Leg." *Scientific American*, October 4, 1862, 224.

Ingraham, Chris. *Enabling the Human Spirit: The J. E. Hanger Story.* Tarentum, Pa.: Word Association, 2003.

Jewett, Benjamin W. *Jewett's Patent Artificial Leg Company.* Washington, D.C.: McGill & Witherow, 1865.

Jewett, George B. *The Salem Leg, under the Patronage of the United States Government for the Use of the Army and Navy.* Salem, Mass.: Salem Leg, 1864.

Laws of Congress in Regard to Taxes, Currency and Conscription, Passed February 1864. Richmond: James E. Goode, 1864.

Laws of the United States Relating to Internal Revenue, Comprising the Act of June 30, 1864, as Amended by Subsequent Acts, Including the Act of March 20, 1867. Washington, D.C.: Government Printing Office, 1867.

Lee, Fitzhugh. "The Death of Colonel Dahlgren." *Historical Magazine*, April 1870, 256–58.

Leggett, M. D. *Subject-Matter Index of Patents for Inventions Issued by the United States Patent Office from 1790 to 1873, Inclusive*, 3 vols. Washington, D.C.: Government Printing Office, 1874.

Lewis, Robert M. Report of the General Superintendent of the Philadelphia Branch of the U.S. Sanitary Commission, to the Executive Committee, January 1st, 1866. Philadelphia: King & Baird, 1866.

Lincoln, Marvin. *Lincoln's Patent Artificial Arm.* New York, 1865.

Little, Henry F. W. *The Seventh Regiment New Hampshire Volunteers in the War of the Rebellion.* Concord, N.H.: Ira C. Evans, 1896.

MacDonald, Joseph, Jr. "The History of Artificial Limbs." *American Journal of Surgery* 19 (October 1905): 76–80.

"Maimed Soldiers." *Medical and Surgical Reporter* 11 (March 19, 1864), 184–85.

Marks, A. A. *Marks' Patent Artificial Limbs, with India Rubber Hands and Feet.* New York: William B. Smyth, 1865.

Marks, George E. *Manual of Artificial Limbs.* New York: A. A. Marks, 1908.

———. *A Treatise on Artificial Limbs with Rubber Hands and Feet* . . . New York: A. A. Marks, 1896.

———. *A Treatise on Marks' Patent Artificial Limbs with Rubber Hands and Feet.* New York: A. A. Marks, 1888.

Marsh, S. N. *A Plain and Popular Explanation of the Nature, Varieties, Treatment and Cure of Hernia, or Rupture.* New York: John Medole, 1860.

Maxwell, David G. "The Two Brothers." In *Histories of the Several Regiments and Battalions from North Carolina in the Great War 1861–65,* edited by Walter Clark, 4:404–6. Goldsboro, N.C.: Nash Brothers, 1901.

McCawley, Patrick J. *Artificial Limbs for Confederate Soldiers.* Columbia: South Carolina Department of Archives and History, 1992.

McDaid, Jennifer Davis. "'How a One-Legged Rebel Lives': Confederate Veterans and Artificial Limbs in Virginia." In *Artificial Parts, Practical Lives: Modern Histories of Prosthetics,* edited by Katherine Ott, David Serlin, and Stephen Mihm, 119–43. New York: New York University Press, 2002.

McPherson, James M. *For Cause and Comrades: Why Men Fought in the Civil War.* New York: Oxford University Press, 1997.

Medical and Surgical History of the War of the Rebellion. Washington, D.C.: Government Printing Office, 1875–85.

"Medical Intelligence." *Boston Medical and Surgical Journal* 71 (October 6, 1864): 208.

Mihm, Stephen. "'A Limb Which Shall Be Presentable in Polite Society': Prosthetic Technologies in the Nineteenth Century." In *Artificial Parts, Practical Lives: Modern Histories of Prosthetics,* edited by Katherine Ott, David Serlin, and Stephen Mihm, 282–99. New York: New York University Press, 2002.

Military Service Records: A Select Catalog of National Archives Microfilm Publications. Washington, D.C.: National Archives and Records Administration, 1985.

Minor, James A. "Report on Artificial Limbs." In *Bulletin of the New York Academy of Medicine, from January 1860 to October 1862,* 163–79. New York: William Wood, 1862.

Monroe and Gardiner's Imperishable Raw Hide Limbs, Patented March 15 and October 11, 1864, and July 25, 1865. New York: Macdonald & Stone, 1866.

Moore, Albert Burton. *Conscription and Conflict in the Confederacy.* Columbia: University of South Carolina Press, 1996.

Munden, Kenneth W., and Henry Putney Beers. *The Union: A Guide to Federal Archives Relating to the Civil War*. Washington, D.C.: National Archives and Records Administration, 1986.

New York City Directory, for 1842 and 1843. New York: John Doggett Jr., 1842.

New York City Directory, 1868-'69. New York: A. B. Taylor [1869?].

"Obituary: D. Willard Bliss." *Medical and Surgical Reporter* 60 (March 9, 1889): 318.

Obituary Record of Graduates of Amherst College, for the Academical Year Ending June 30, 1886. Amherst, Mass.: J. E. Williams, 1886.

Officer, Lawrence H. "Dollar-Pound Exchange Rate from 1791." MeasuringWorth 2008, http://www.measuringworth.org/exchangepound, accessed March 1, 2010.

Orr, James L. *Message No. 1 of His Excellency Gov. J. L. Orr, with Accompanying Documents. Prepared for the Called Session of the Legislature, July, 1868*. Columbia, S.C.: Phoenix Book and Job Power, 1868.

Ott, Katherine. "The Sum of Its Parts: An Introduction to Modern Histories of Prosthetics." In *Artificial Parts, Practical Lives: Modern Histories of Prosthetics*, edited by Katherine Ott, David Serlin, and Stephen Mihm, 1–42. New York: New York University Press, 2002.

Palmer, B. Frank. "Infringements—Caution." *Bane and Antidote*, no. 8 (January 1859): 15–17.

———. *The Palmer Arm and Leg: Adopted for the U.S. Army and Navy, by the Surgeon-General, U.S.A. and by the Chief of the Bureau of Medicine and Surgery, U.S.N.* Philadelphia [1865?].

———. *The Palmer Arm and Leg: Correspondence with the Surgeon General U.S.A. and the Chief of Bureau of Medicine and Surgery U.S.N. with Letters from Eminent Surgeons, and a Communication from B. Frank Palmer to the Board of Surgeons Convened to Decide on the Best Patent Artificial Limbs to be Adopted for Use by the Army and Navy of the U.S.* Philadelphia: C. Sherman & Son, 1862.

———. "Palmer's Artificial Leg in London." *Boston Medical and Surgical Journal* 45 (August 6, 1851): 18–22.

———. "Palmer's Artificial Limbs." *Boston Medical and Surgical Journal* 37 (December 9, 1847): 375–77.

———. *Report of the Great National Benefaction: Seven Thousand Patent Limbs Given to the Mutilated Heroes of the Great War*. Philadelphia: Sherman & Co., 1868.

———. *Steps*. N.p. [1874?].

———. *Will the American Government Present an Artificial Arm (Not a "Clutch") to the Mutilated American Soldier?* N.p., 1863.

"Palmer's Artificial Leg." *Boston Medical and Surgical Journal* 60 (February 3, 1859): 26–27.

"Palmer's Artificial Limbs." *Scientific American*, February 26, 1859, 208.

Papers Relating to Foreign Affairs, Accompanying the Annual Message of the President to the First Session Thirty-Ninth Congress, pt. 1. Washington, D.C.: Government Printing Office, 1866.

Papers Relating to Foreign Affairs, Accompanying the Annual Message of the President to the Second Session Thirty-Eighth Congress, pt. 2. Washington, D.C.: Government Printing Office, 1865.

Pasquina, Paul F., Charles R. Scovill, Brian Belnap, and Rory A. Cooper. "Introduction: Developing a System of Care for the Combat Amputee." In *Care of the Combat Amputee*, edited by Paul F. Pasquina and Rory A. Cooper, 1–18. Washington, D.C.: Office of the Surgeon General, 2009.

Pollard, Edward A. *Life of Jefferson Davis, with a Secret History of the Southern Confederacy, Gathered "Behind the Scenes in Richmond."* Philadelphia: National, 1869.

Porter, Felicia G. Circular, April 18, 1866. *De Bow's Review*, n.s., 1 (June 1866): 664.

Potts, James. "Mr. Potts, on the Means of Supplying the Loss of Amputated Limbs." *Medical and Physical Journal* 5 (March 1801): 277–78.

"Proceedings of the Second Confederate Congress, December 15, 1864, to March 18, 1865." *Southern Historical Society Papers*, n.s., 14 (1959).

"Progress of Medicine." *Nashville Journal of Medicine and Surgery* 3 (June 1868): 521–40.

Reznick, Jeffrey S., Jeff Gambel, and Alan J. Hawk. "Historical Perspectives on the Care of Service Members with Limb Amputations." In *Care of the Combat Amputee*, edited by Paul F. Pasquina and Rory A. Cooper, 19–40. Washington, D.C.: Office of the Surgeon General, 2009.

Rhodes, Rufus R. *Annual Report of the Commissioner of Patents*. Richmond: Confederate States Patent Office, 1865.

———. *Report of the Commissioner of Patents*. Richmond: Confederate States Patent Office, 1864.

Robert, Charles E. *Nashville and Her Trade for 1870*. Nashville: Roberts & Purvis, 1870.

Schmidt, James M. "A Multiplicity of Ingenious Articles." In *Years of Change and Suffering: Modern Perspectives on Civil War Medicine*, edited by James M. Schmidt and Guy R Hasegawa, 37–55. Roseville, Minn.: Edinborough, 2009.

Schultz, Duane. *The Dahlgren Affair: Terror and Conspiracy in the Civil War*. New York: W. W. Norton, 1998.

Schwab, John Christopher. *The Confederate States of America, 1861–1865: A Financial and Industrial History of the South during the Civil War*. New York: Charles Scribner's Sons, 1901.

Selpho, William. *The Best Substitutes for Natural Limbs, the World of Science Has Even Invented!* New York [1863?].

Smith, Henry H. *The Principles and Practice of Surgery . . .* , vol. 2. Philadelphia: Lippincott, 1863.

Stansbury, Charles F. *Argument in Behalf of the Extension of the Patent of B. Frank. Palmer, for an Improvement in Artificial Legs, Dated November 4th, 1846*. N.p., 1860.

———. *Testimony in Behalf of the Extension of the Patent of B. Frank. Palmer, for an Improvement in Artificial Legs, Dated November 4th, 1846*. N.p. [1860?].

Stillé, Charles J. *History of the United States Sanitary Commission, Being the General Report of Its Work during the War of the Rebellion*. Philadelphia: J. B. Lippincott, 1866.

Sutherland, Charles. *Report of the Surgeon-General of the Army to the Secretary of War for the Fiscal Year Ending June 30, 1892*. Washington, D.C.: Government Printing Office, 1892.

Tax-Payer's Manual: Containing the Direct and Excise Taxes. . . . New York: D. Appleton, 1863.

Taylor, William F. *Annual Report of the Auditor of Public Accounts [Virginia] for the Fiscal Year Ending September 30, 1872.* Richmond: R. F. Walker, 1872.

———. *Report of the Auditor of Public Accounts [Virginia] for the Fiscal Year Ending September 30, 1873.* Richmond: R. F. Walker, 1873.

Tenth Exhibition of the Massachusetts Charitable Mechanic Association, at Fanueil and Quincy Halls, in the City of Boston, September and October, 1865. Boston: Wright & Potter, 1865.

Transactions of the American Institute of the City of New-York, for the Year 1850. Albany: Charles Van Benthuysen, 1851.

Transactions of the American Institute of the City of New-York, for the Year 1857. Albany: Charles Van Benthuysen, 1858.

Transactions of the N.Y. State Agricultural Society, with an Abstract of the Proceedings of the County Agricultural Societies. Albany: Charles Van Benthuysen, 1859.

Trow's New York City Directory, vol. 78. New York: John F. Trow, 1865.

Trow's New York City Directory, vol. 79. New York: John F. Trow, 1866.

U.S. Sanitary Commission. *The Soldier's Friend.* Philadelphia: Perkinpine & Higgins, 1865.

Wales, Philip S. *Mechanical Therapeutics. A Practical Treatise on Surgical Apparatus, Alliances, and Elementary Operations.* . . . Philadelphia: Henry C. Lea, 1867.

War of the Rebellion: A Compilation of the Official Records of the Union and Confederate Armies. Washington, D.C.: Government Printing Office, 1880–1901.

Warren, Edward. *Report of the Surgeon General of North Carolina.* Raleigh: Surgeon General's Office, 1864.

"The Week." *American Medical Times,* December 21, 1861, 409–10.

"The Week." *American Medical Times,* October 18, 1862, 220.

Wegner, Ansley Herring. *Phantom Pain: North Carolina's Artificial-Limbs Program for Confederate Veterans.* Raleigh: North Carolina Department of Cultural Resources, 2004.

Weidenmier, Marc D. "Turning Points in the U.S. Civil War: Views from the Grayback Market." *Southern Economic Journal* 68 (April 2002): 875–90.

Welles, Gideon. Report of the Secretary of the Navy, in *Message from the President of the United States to the Two Houses of Congress, at the Commencement of the First Session of the Thirty-Ninth Congress.* . . . Washington, DC: Government Printing Office, 1866.

Whitson, J. C. "Letters from the South." *Scientific American,* June 8, 1861, 358.

Williamson, James J. *Mosby's Rangers: A Record of the Operations of the Forty-Third Battalion Virginia Cavalry.* New York: Ralph B. Kenyon, 1896.

Wilson, Harold S. *Confederate Industry.* Jackson: University Press of Mississippi, 2002.

Wilson's New York City Copartnership Directory, for 1866-'67. New York: John F. Trow, 1866.

Winthrop, W., ed., *A Digest of Opinions of the Judge Advocates General of the Army with Notes.* Washington, D.C.: Government Printing Office, 1895.

Wise, Stephen R. *Lifeline of the Confederacy: Blockade Running during the Civil War.* Columbia: University of South Carolina Press, 1988.

Wittenberg, Eric J. *Like a Meteor Blazing Brightly: The Short but Controversial Life of Colonel Ulric Dahlgren.* Roseville, Minn.: Edinborough, 2009.

Woodward, C. Vann, ed. *Mary Chesnut's Civil War.* New Haven: Yale University Press, 1981.

INDEX

Weston, James W., 85, 91; self-pro-
motion, 16, 74, 109n7, gallery (17th
image); and U.S. limbs program, 39,
110n11
whalebone, 13, 85
Wharncliffe, Lord, 64–65
Whelan, William, 22, 25
Wigfall, Louis T., 68
Wilcox, O. D., 11, 12, 34, 90, 91
Williams (shoe manufacturer), 55
Wilmington, N.C., 90

Winkley Artificial Limb Company, 78,
108n16
wood: as limb constituent, 12, 14,
52, 54, 71; in peg legs, 48; poplar,
54; seasoned, 12, 55; willow, 9, 12,
104n17
Wood, Robert Crooke, 26
wounds, 1–2

Yerger, George W., 13, 16, 49, 91; limb
made by Matlack, 17, 30, 39, 87

Guy R. Hasegawa is an editor for the *American Journal of Health-System Pharmacy* in Bethesda, Maryland. In addition to his numerous articles on Civil War medicine, he contributed to and coedited *Years of Change and Suffering: Modern Perspectives on Civil War Medicine.*